THE MEDICINE-FREE,
ILLNESS-FREE SERIES

HOPED PROTOCOL

Five Key Nutrients for Lifelong Health

Forest Yin, DAOM, L.Ac.

Ashi Healing Publishing

First Edition: May 2025

Published by Ashi Healing

www.AshiHealing.com

Paperback ISBN: 978-1-967735-10-5

eBook ISBN: 978-1-967735-11-2

Printed in the United States of America

Medical Disclaimer:

This book is for informational purposes only and is not intended as medical advice. The author and publisher assume no responsibility for how the information is used. Readers should consult a healthcare professional before making any health-related decisions.

Foreword

Nature is the origin of life, the origin of healing, and remains a guiding force in human well-being. Long before modern science developed medicine in laboratories, nature provided everything the human body needed to survive, and to sustain life. The food we eat, the herbs we gather, the minerals beneath our feet, and the sun above us are all part of an intelligent and interconnected system that has long nourished and supported the human body.

This truth has been known across cultures for thousands of years, and it is echoed in sacred texts. In the Book of Genesis, the Garden of Eden was described as a paradise where "every tree that is pleasant to the sight and good for food" was made available to humankind (Genesis 2:9). Some scholars believe this refers not only to nourishment, but also to the ability to contribute to human well-being. It becomes even more clear in Ezekiel 47:12: "The fruit thereof shall be for meat, and the leaf thereof for medicine."

Somewhere along the way, modern culture drifted from this wisdom. Many now believe that healing must come through synthetic drugs, surgeries, or man-made interventions, forgetting that the foundation of human health has always been rooted in nature. But what if well-being isn't only about medical breakthroughs, but also about reconnecting with what has always been available to us?

What if the body doesn't need to be forced to function differently, but simply supported, nourished, balanced, and reminded of what it already knows? What if illness is not the enemy, but a signal that we've fallen out of balance, and out of sync with nature?

This is not to dismiss the value of conventional medicine. We are deeply grateful for its life-saving capabilities in emergencies and acute care. But when it comes to supporting long-term vitality and encouraging balance, it may be time to return to the source.

In addition to thousands of years of lived wisdom, modern science is now exploring the potential of many natural approaches. What was once viewed as "alternative" is now increasingly recognized as part of a broader wellness conversation.

This book, and the entire *Medicine-Free, Illness-Free Series*, is rooted in this truth:

Nature not only gave us life. Many believe it holds the power to support our well-being. And many of these natural approaches are now being studied and better understood through science.

Healing is not something we must force or fear. It is something we can encourage, by gently supporting the body, naturally.

Dr. Forest Yin, DAOM, L.Ac.

Author, *The Medicine-Free, Illness-Free Series*

Founder, Ashi Healing and Acupuncture Inc.

Important Disclaimer

The supplements, therapies, and natural approaches discussed in *The Medicine-Free, Illness-Free Series* are intended to support general wellness and the body's natural balance. They are not intended to diagnose, treat, cure, or prevent any disease and have not been evaluated by the U.S. Food and Drug Administration (FDA).

These books are provided for educational purposes only and are not a substitute for professional medical advice, diagnosis, or treatment. Always consult your physician or a licensed healthcare provider before starting any new supplement, therapy, or wellness routine, especially if you are pregnant, nursing, have a medical condition, or are taking medications.

The content in this series is informed by two sources: summaries of available scientific research, presented as "Science-Informed Solution Benefits", and aggregated user feedback, presented as "Customer-Reported Solution Benefits". These are intended to inform and inspire, but they reflect general patterns, not guarantees. Individual results will vary.

The phrase *"Medicine-Free, Illness-Free"* reflects a natural wellness philosophy and is not a medical claim or promise of outcome.

By reading this book, you agree to take full responsibility for your personal health choices and to seek guidance from qualified health professionals when needed.

Contents

Preface

Do you feel like you've tried everything—medications, conventional treatments, even supplements—yet still struggle with fatigue, discomfort, brain fog, or other daily wellness concerns?

If so, you're not alone.

Many people today are turning to nature-based solutions, not as replacements for essential medical care, but as gentle, sustainable ways to support their overall well-being.

The rise in chronic health challenges reflects this shift. According to the CDC, over 60% of U.S. adults live with at least one chronic health condition, and more than 40% manage two or more. More than 40% of school-aged children in the United States are reported to have at least one ongoing wellness concern, rising sharply in recent years.

At the same time, modern habits, nutrient-depleted diets, environmental stressors, and sedentary routines, have created a disconnect between how we live and what the body truly needs to stay resilient. For many, conventional solutions haven't fully addressed these patterns, leaving people still searching for support that feels both effective and sustainable.

That's what *The Medicine-Free, Illness-Free Series* is here to explore.

This series introduces practical, natural options that may help support energy, digestion, sleep, focus, mood, and more, without requiring major lifestyle changes or complicated routines.

It doesn't reject conventional medicine. It expands your toolkit. While modern treatments often focus on managing symptoms in the short term, natural health practices are designed to work more gradually, supporting the body's natural rhythms over time. Many people are rediscovering how ancient practices and modern science can work together, not in opposition, to create a more balanced, resilient life.

The Medicine-Free, Illness-Free Series is built on two foundational pillars:

Science-Informed Solution Benefits: exploring what modern research says about the potential benefits associated with each supplement or therapy

Customer-Reported Solution Benefits: drawn from thousands of real-world user feedback to highlight what people most often experience in practice, including common benefit themes, typical use case patterns, and key user insights.

By combining scientific research with traditional use and real-world user feedback, each volume empowers you to make informed decisions, grounded in both evidence and everyday reality.

Each book in the series focuses on one category of natural therapies. Whether you're exploring Herbal Therapy, Mushroom Therapy, Amino Acid support, Animal Organ Supplements, Grounding, the HOPED Protocol, or detoxification, the goal is the same: to offer trusted solutions that fit easily into your life, simply, naturally, and sustainably.

You don't need to overhaul your lifestyle or commit to an elaborate health plan. You can begin right where you are. Even one small step, a single herb, nutrient, or daily practice, can help you create a rhythm of care that supports your body more naturally over time.

Preface

While no approach guarantees results, many people have found these natural strategies helpful in supporting comfort, energy, focus, and overall vitality. This series was created to help you explore those tools with clarity and confidence, without pressure or complexity.

This volume focuses on the HOPED Protocol, offering practical insight into five foundational pillars—High-fiber foods, Omega-3s and Antioxidants, Probiotics, Enzymes, and Vitamin D—that help support long-term health. You'll learn about each element through both research and real-world perspectives, so you can decide what feels right for your journey.

Thank you for beginning this exploration.

Let's move forward, one natural step at a time.

The Medicine-Free, Illness-Free Series

The Medicine-Free, Illness-Free Series is your go-to resource for practical, research-informed natural strategies that are easy to apply. Each volume focuses on a single modality or system—herbs, mushrooms, organ supplements, amino acids, grounding, detox, and more—offering clear guidance to help you choose what works best for you.

Together, the 10 books provide a comprehensive yet flexible wellness framework that supports both daily health maintenance and targeted support. Here's a brief overview of what you'll find in each book:

The Medicine-Free, Illness-Free Series: Why Natural Health Is the Future

Explore why millions of people are turning to nature-aligned strategies to support their wellness. This foundational volume introduces the core science and philosophy behind natural approaches to health, and how they may support your sense of balance, vitality, and overall well-being.

The Medicine-Free, Illness-Free Series: Herbal Therapy

Learn how the world's most time-tested plants may support digestion, energy, relaxation, immune strength, and more. Discover practical ways to include them in your routine and how to choose herbs that match your personal needs and constitution.

The Medicine-Free, Illness-Free Series: Mushroom Therapy

Discover the unique compounds found in medicinal mushrooms that may support immunity, cognitive function, and stress resilience. This book explains how to use mushrooms such as Reishi, Lion's Mane, and Cordyceps in a daily supplement.

The Medicine-Free, Illness-Free Series: Animal Organ Therapy

Explore how nutrient-dense organ supplements, like liver, heart, and kidney, may provide highly bioavailable vitamins, minerals, and peptides. Learn how these traditional foods may support foundational wellness in areas like energy, endurance, and metabolic balance.

The Medicine-Free, Illness-Free Series: Amino Acid Therapy

Uncover the role of amino acids, the building blocks of life, in supporting mood, focus, muscle strength, and nervous system health. This volume shows how targeted amino acid support may help restore clarity, resilience, and emotional well-being.

The Medicine-Free, Illness-Free Series: HOPED Protocol

Learn the five foundational nutrient categories—High Fiber, Omega-3s & Antioxidants, Probiotics, Enzymes, and Vitamin D—and how to implement them as a core wellness strategy. HOPED is simple, actionable, and designed for everyday consistency.

The Medicine-Free, Illness-Free Series: Detoxification Therapy

Discover a gentle, nature-based approach to support your body's natural detoxification processes, promote balance, and encourage overall vitality using simple, practical techniques.

The Medicine-Free, Illness-Free Series: Grounding Therapy

Explore the science and practice of grounding (earthing), the natural process of reconnecting with the Earth's electrical field. Learn how this subtle practice may help support nervous system regulation, sleep quality, and emotional balance.

The Medicine-Free, Illness-Free Series: Diet, Lifestyle and Emotional Well-being

While drastic changes are not required, this volume introduces simple habits that promote long-term balance, covering food, movement, sleep, and emotional self-regulation in a way that aligns with the rest of your natural health plan.

The Medicine-Free, Illness-Free Series: Integrative Therapies for Everyday Health

This final volume brings together insights from the entire series, offering user-reported tools to help support everyday wellness goals, such as energy, digestion, sleep, immunity, and emotional resilience. It serves as a cross-reference for applying the therapies in complementary ways, helping you navigate your health journey with clarity and confidence.

Meet Dr. Forest Yin, DAOM, L.Ac.

Professionally known as Forest Yin, my official name is Jie Yin, while also known as 尹明杰 in the Chinese speaking communities.

For most of my professional life, I was known as a high-tech executive, problem-solver, and innovator in information security and technologies. In leadership roles at Oracle, Schwab, and Wells Fargo, I developed and managed advanced security solutions, ensuring stability, efficiency, and high performance in a fast-paced, high-stakes environment.

But after work, I was deeply immersed in another world, the science of natural health.

My journey into Traditional Chinese Medicine (TCM) began in college, when I first studied the *Huang Di Nei Jing (Yellow Emperor's Classic of Internal Medicine)* alongside my Physics degree. While excelling in my tech career, I continued to research, experiment, and apply natural healing principles, seeking ways to optimize health, energy, and resilience, not just for myself, but for those around me.

Recognizing the profound impact of natural medicine on long-term health and performance, I pursued formal training, becoming a Licensed Acupuncturist (L.Ac.) in 2018 and earning my Doctorate in Acupuncture and Oriental Medicine (DAOM) in 2019. Since then, I have supported individuals around the world in improving their vitality, resilience, and sense of well-being through natural methods. This led me to found Ashi Healing and Acupuncture Inc. and become a Professor and Doctoral Advisor at the University of East-West Medicine, where I mentor future practitioners in the art of TCM.

Applying Systems Thinking to Health & Healing

In high-tech, solving problems requires understanding systems, identifying vulnerabilities, and optimizing performance. I apply the same mindset to health. Instead of treating symptoms, I look at the root cause, like debugging a system. Instead of temporary fixes, I focus on long-term balance and resilience, like designing sustainable architecture. Instead of pharmaceutical dependency, I seek efficient, natural approaches that support function and balance gently, without the common side effects associated with conventional options, like optimizing system performance.

While many of my colleagues in the tech and finance industries thrived in their careers, I also saw the toll of chronic stress, burnout, autoimmune conditions, and lifestyle-related illnesses. Like many professionals, they pushed their limits, until their bodies pushed back. This is where natural approaches can make a difference.

A Philosophy Rooted in Balance & Natural Healing

At Ashi Healing, my approach complements conventional care by focusing on identifying underlying imbalances and supporting the body's natural self-regulation through Traditional Chinese Medicine and holistic strategies.

The name "Ashi (阿是)" comes from a fundamental concept in Chinese medicine, that moment of realization when healing feels real. In Chinese, "Ashi" means "Ahh, Yes!", the instant when your body recognizes exactly what it needs. This guiding philosophy shapes everything I do, from acupuncture to natural health solutions.

Through the precise use of Chinese Herbal Medicine and modern whole-food-based natural supplements like herbs and mushrooms, I have helped individuals support their energy and balance naturally, using simple, sustainable tools that complement or reduce the need for pharmaceutical interventions when appropriate.

My mission is simple: to help people pursue wellness and resilience, naturally and sustainably.

Integrating Ancient Wisdom with Modern Innovation

Chinese Herbal Medicine has been refined for thousands of years. But today, we can take it further, combining ancient wisdom with modern research and a strategic, data-driven approach to health optimization.

At Ashi Healing, I personalize each protocol based on the individual's needs, whether it's boosting energy, reducing stress, improving cognitive function, or addressing chronic health concerns. Many of the people I work with are busy professionals seeking practical, time-efficient strategies to support their health without disrupting their demanding schedules.

Looking for More Information and Support

To learn more about my personalized approach to Chinese Herbal Therapy and whole-food-based supplements, visit AshiHealing.com. You'll find additional resources and simple ways to take the next step in your healing journey, whenever you're ready.

And remember, this book is just one part of *The Medicine-Free, Illness-Free Series.* Each volume explores a different pillar of natural healing, from herbs and mushrooms to amino acids, detoxification, and grounding, offering you a complete path to support your balance and well-being through nature-based strategies.

A Science-Backed, Real-World Tested Method

In *The Medicine-Free, Illness-Free Series*, we introduce a unique, structured method for exploring natural supplements, one that blends scientific insight with real-world observations. Rather than relying solely on clinical studies or anecdotal reports, we combine both perspectives to give you a well-rounded, user-friendly understanding of each natural solution.

This balanced approach helps answer the most important questions: What does science suggest about this supplement's potential? What are people actually experiencing when they use it? Which health goals do people turn to it for most often?

Our method reflects a commitment to transparency, education, and practicality, so you can explore these natural options with clarity and confidence.

Our Four-Part Analysis Method

1. Science-Informed Solution Benefits

We begin by reviewing peer-reviewed studies, traditional usage patterns, and emerging scientific literature to understand the possible mechanisms and effects of each supplement. This provides a foundation of what is known, hypothesized, or being actively researched, offering a science-informed perspective to guide your exploration.

2. Customer-Reported Solution Benefits

We analyze large sets of customer reviews from publicly available platforms to understand how these supplements are being used in daily life. This includes what benefits people say they notice most often and how they describe their experiences.

Our focus is on patterns of what users commonly report, rather than isolated stories. This real-world layer helps connect the theory to practical, everyday outcomes.

3. Use Case Patterns & Feedback Insights

Within the customer-reported section, we highlight:

Use Case Patterns Observed – What kinds of goals or wellness concerns people most commonly use each supplement for.

Feedback Insights – How users describe the impact in their own words, including sentiment, language tone, and satisfaction cues.

Most Reported Benefits – A percentage-based summary showing which benefits are mentioned most often in reviews.

This structured summary lets you see what real people are using the supplement for, and how frequently those benefits are reported.

4. No Brand Promotion—Just Trusted Guidance

This series does not promote specific products or brands. Instead, we offer education and a decision-making framework. For those looking for high-quality sources, recommended supplement types and vetted options are available at AshiHealing.com.

Why This Method Matters

In today's crowded supplement market, it can be hard to separate hype from helpful information. That's why we created this approach, to empower you with insights drawn from scientific research, real-world usage patterns and satisfaction trends, and clear summaries that help you compare options and set expectations

You won't find exaggerated claims or one-size-fits-all solutions here. Instead, you'll find a practical, transparent method that reflects how real people are exploring natural wellness, with science as a guide and personal experience as a reference.

Whether you're considering herbs, mushrooms, amino acids, or other supplements, this method gives you a safe and structured way to learn how others are using these tools, and how they might fit into your own wellness journey.

A Personal Commitment from Dr. Forest Yin

Every approach, strategy, and supplement featured in *The Medicine-Free, Illness-Free Series* has been personally explored. Before sharing any recommendations with clients or readers, I take the time to experience it myself, observing how it affects energy, mood, sleep, digestion, and focus.

This hands-on approach allows me to understand each therapy not just through science, or just through other people's experiences. It adds a personal layer of insight to the research and user-reported feedback that shape this series.

My goal is simple: to help you find natural, sustainable solutions that feel doable, helpful, and aligned with how lasting wellness begins, by reconnecting with your body's own rhythms and innate intelligence.

HOPED – What Is It?

As you continue your journey toward greater health and vitality, the foundational practices introduced in earlier volumes—herbal remedies, mushroom therapies, animal organ supplements, and amino acid supplementation—have already equipped you with effective tools for nourishment and self-care. These therapies offer concentrated nutrients in their most bioavailable forms, helping support the body at a cellular level and encouraging a balanced gut microbiome.

Building upon that strong foundation, the HOPED protocol introduces a focused, five-part strategy for optimizing wellness. HOPED stands for High Fiber, Omega-3 and Antioxidants, Probiotics, Enzymes, and Vitamin D. Each pillar has been thoughtfully selected to complement the core therapies you've already explored, helping to bridge nutritional gaps and enhance the body's natural ability to maintain balance and resilience.

One of the guiding principles behind HOPED is the emphasis on natural, food-based sources whenever possible. Unlike synthetic isolates, which may vary in absorption or compatibility, nutrients from whole-food or nature-identical sources are typically more easily absorbed and utilized by the body. Choosing these cleaner, more compatible forms allows for a gentler, more supportive approach to supplementation.

In the chapters that follow, you'll explore how each of these five components can contribute to a more complete and integrated wellness plan:

High Fiber: Discover how dietary fibers such as psyllium husk may support gut health, help stabilize blood sugar levels and assist in maintaining cardiovascular wellness. Fiber forms the cornerstone of digestive support, aiding in toxin removal and enhancing nutrient absorption.

Omega-3 and Antioxidants: Learn how Omega-3 fatty acids and antioxidants may work together to help manage inflammatory responses, reduce oxidative stress, and support cellular integrity. We'll explore key sources including fish oil, krill oil, algae oil, CoQ10, resveratrol, and Shilajit, a naturally occurring mineral resin valued for its antioxidant content and trace minerals.

Probiotics: Understand the role of beneficial bacteria in digestive balance, nutrient metabolism, and immune function. You'll see how the previous therapies in this series help create a favorable environment for probiotics, and how these microorganisms can further support your system's resilience.

Enzymes: While many organ-based supplements naturally provide enzymatic activity, targeted enzyme support, including Betaine HCL, may help improve digestion and nutrient uptake, especially for those who experience sluggish digestion or low stomach acid levels.

Vitamin D: Widely recognized for its importance in bone health and immune balance, Vitamin D is also involved in hormonal and metabolic processes. Many people benefit from targeted supplementation, especially in seasons or regions with limited sun exposure. We'll look at natural sources such as cod liver oil, fish eggs, and high-quality D3 options.

By integrating the HOPED framework into your ongoing routine, you can reinforce key areas of health, respond to specific needs, and promote a more complete sense of well-being. This streamlined yet powerful protocol offers a clear next step in your self-care journey, allowing you to approach health from multiple angles, gently, naturally, and effectively.

What to Expect in This Book

In this guide, we explore the HOPED Protocol—a practical, five-part framework built around key nutritional supports: High Fiber, Omega-3 and Antioxidants, Probiotics, Enzymes, and Vitamin D. These core components are often overlooked, yet they play a crucial role in supporting digestion, immunity, energy, and overall vitality.

Each chapter focuses on one of these five pillars using a dual-lens approach that blends scientific insight with real-world experience. The goal is to help you understand how these widely used supplements may fit into your wellness strategy with clarity and confidence.

Here's what each section includes:

Science-Informed Solution Benefits

Each chapter begins with an overview of what current research says about the nutrient's role in supporting key body systems. You'll learn how it functions, where it shows promise, and what the evidence suggests—without making specific health claims.

Customer-Reported Solution Benefits

We analyzed thousands of verified product reviews to better understand how people use and respond to each supplement. This section includes:

Use Case Patterns Observed: Common reasons people take each supplement, such as digestive support, energy, mood, or immune health.

Feedback Insights: How users describe their experience and how the supplement fits into their daily routines.

Most Reported Benefits: A summary table showing the most frequently mentioned outcomes, with percentages from large-scale review analysis.

Solutions for Everyday Health Goals

At the end of the book, you'll find a reference section that maps common wellness goals—like fatigue, digestive discomfort, or sleep support—to the HOPED components most frequently associated with those goals. This resource is educational, not diagnostic, and is meant to support informed decision-making.

Whether your focus is energy, digestion, mood, or immune resilience, this book offers trusted guidance rooted in both science and lived experience. By understanding how the HOPED Protocol works in real life, you'll be better equipped to take simple, effective steps toward greater balance and vitality.

.

High Fiber

Fiber is one of the most essential, yet frequently overlooked, components of a healthy diet. Despite widespread awareness of its importance, most people still fall significantly short of the daily recommended intake. The consequences of this shortfall ripple across multiple areas of health, affecting digestion, energy, weight balance, and overall vitality.

A Modern Deficiency Rooted in Modern Habits

Historically, human diets were rich in fiber due to the abundance of unprocessed, plant-based foods. Fruits, vegetables, seeds, roots, and whole grains naturally provided the bulk that kept the digestive system moving and supported internal balance. However, in today's fast-paced world, many of those foods have been replaced by modern conveniences. Pre-packaged meals, refined snacks, sugary drinks, and fast food have become dietary staples. These items are often stripped of their fiber content during processing, leaving behind calories with little nutritional value.

Even when individuals make a conscious effort to eat "healthy," their meals may still lack the consistent fiber levels needed to support digestion and long-term wellness. Salads, smoothies, and occasional servings of vegetables may not be enough to reach the ideal fiber threshold, especially when meals are irregular or portion sizes are limited.

According to national dietary surveys, the average American consumes only about 15 grams of fiber per day, while the recommended amount is 25 to 38 grams depending on age and sex. This shortfall is known as the "fiber gap," and it is a widespread public health concern that can have real, cumulative effects on well-being over time.

Why Fiber Matters More Than Most People Realize

Fiber plays a crucial role in many foundational processes in the body. It helps support regular bowel movements by adding bulk and promoting motility. It contributes to the removal of waste and byproducts, supports gut microbiome diversity, and helps maintain healthy blood sugar and lipid levels already within normal range. Fiber may also promote a sense of fullness, which can influence appetite regulation in a positive way.

There are two main types of fiber, soluble and insoluble, and both contribute differently to health:

Soluble fiber dissolves in water to form a gel-like substance. It is found in foods like oats, apples, flaxseed, and legumes, and it plays a role in slowing digestion and supporting balanced nutrient absorption.

Insoluble fiber does not dissolve in water. It adds bulk to the stool and supports regular elimination. Sources include whole grains, vegetables, and seeds.

While each type serves a unique function, most whole plant foods contain a combination of both. Unfortunately, the more a food is refined, the more likely it is to be stripped of this important nutritional content.

The Consequences of Too Little Fiber

When fiber intake falls short, the body feels it. Many people who experience occasional constipation, irregular digestion, bloating, or sluggishness may be unknowingly dealing with a fiber deficit. Low fiber diets have also been associated with poor gut microbiome diversity, which is increasingly linked to various aspects of systemic health, including immune resilience and emotional well-being.

Lack of fiber may also contribute to imbalances in blood sugar regulation, as fiber helps slow the absorption of carbohydrates and smooth out energy fluctuations. Over time, a diet consistently low in fiber can create conditions that make it more difficult to maintain a healthy metabolism and digestive rhythm.

While many of these issues can be addressed through dietary improvements, the reality is that most people struggle to make the necessary changes consistently. This is where supplementation becomes both a practical and powerful tool.

The Role of Fiber Supplements in Closing the Gap

For those unable to consistently meet their fiber needs through diet alone, a high-quality fiber supplement can offer an effective solution. Supplements provide a concentrated source of either soluble, insoluble, or combined fiber forms. They are easy to incorporate into daily routines, often requiring nothing more than a glass of water and a few seconds of preparation.

One of the most widely used and well-researched options is Psyllium Husk, a soluble fiber that has been used for decades to support digestive regularity and overall fiber intake. Its gel-forming properties allow it to expand in the digestive tract, providing the bulk and softness needed for easier elimination. Beyond its physical effects, Psyllium has also been shown to help support a healthy internal environment in the gut, especially when consumed consistently as part of a daily wellness regimen.

Fiber supplementation is not a replacement for whole foods, but it can be an incredibly useful addition to a wellness strategy, particularly for busy individuals, picky eaters, or anyone navigating dietary limitations. Whether you're traveling, adjusting to a new meal plan, or simply looking to improve regularity and gut comfort, fiber supplements offer targeted support where it's often needed most.

Laying the Foundation for Better Health

In the chapters that follow, you'll learn more about the science-informed and customer-reported benefits of Psyllium Husk. This supplement has become a cornerstone for many people seeking better digestive health, improved elimination, and a stronger sense of internal balance.

The HOPED Protocol begins here with fiber, because true wellness starts with a well-functioning digestive system. When the gut is supported, the rest of the body is better able to absorb nutrients, eliminate waste, and maintain balance. In many ways, fiber sets the stage for every other therapy in this book to work more effectively.

Let's begin with a closer look at Psyllium Fiber and why it continues to be one of the most trusted tools for bridging the fiber gap in modern life.

Psyllium Fiber

Psyllium fiber, sourced from the husks of *Plantago ovata* seeds, is a naturally occurring soluble fiber that has earned a long-standing reputation for supporting digestive health and overall balance. Used for centuries in traditional wellness practices, psyllium continues to be widely embraced today for its ability to promote regularity and nourish the digestive system in a gentle yet effective way. Its benefits, however, extend far beyond the gut.

One of the most compelling features of psyllium fiber is its ability to form a thick, gel-like substance when mixed with water. This physical property allows it to act as both a bulking agent and a modulator of absorption in the gastrointestinal tract. These effects contribute to a range of supportive functions across digestion, metabolism, and cardiovascular wellness.

In modern life, where low-fiber diets and digestive imbalances are common, psyllium offers a practical, natural approach to helping restore internal balance. Whether used for daily maintenance or as targeted support during periods of dietary disruption, psyllium is valued for its reliability, tolerability, and simplicity. It can be stirred into water, added to smoothies, or taken in capsule form, making it easy to integrate into a wide variety of routines.

Science-Informed Psyllium Fiber Benefits

Scientific studies have explored how psyllium supports key physiological functions and contributes to overall wellness. The benefits listed below reflect findings from peer-reviewed research that describe how psyllium interacts with the digestive and metabolic systems. These mechanisms are not intended to imply treatment of medical conditions, but rather to offer insight into how this fiber operates within the body.

Supports Digestive Regularity

Psyllium's most well-known benefit is its ability to promote healthy, consistent bowel movements. When psyllium absorbs water, it expands and forms a gel that increases stool bulk and softness. This action can support smoother elimination and help individuals maintain regularity, especially when their diet is low in naturally fibrous foods.

Psyllium is often used by individuals who experience occasional constipation or inconsistent digestive patterns. Its gentle nature allows it to work without harsh stimulation, which is why it is frequently preferred over stimulant-based alternatives. It may also assist in maintaining comfort during periods of dietary transition or travel.

Promotes Cardiovascular Wellness Through Cholesterol Regulation

Research suggests that psyllium may support cardiovascular health by assisting the body in maintaining healthy cholesterol levels already within a normal range. It does this by binding to bile acids in the intestines, which are then eliminated through the stool. The body must use cholesterol to produce more bile acids, which may result in a reduction in circulating low-density lipoprotein (LDL) levels.

This process does not appear to significantly affect high-density lipoprotein (HDL) levels, which are considered beneficial. When incorporated into a fiber-rich diet, psyllium may be a useful addition to support heart health, especially in individuals monitoring their lipid profiles as part of a broader wellness strategy.

Helps Support Blood Sugar Balance

Psyllium's gel-forming behavior slows the digestion and absorption of carbohydrates, which can contribute to more stable post-meal blood sugar levels. This effect may help support glycemic balance and reduce the sharp fluctuations in energy that sometimes occur after meals high in simple carbohydrates.

For individuals who are mindful of their carbohydrate intake or who are managing blood sugar stability as part of a nutritional plan, psyllium can provide an added layer of support. It is most effective when consumed alongside meals or mixed into beverages with other food sources.

Contributes to Healthy Weight Management

Satiety, or the feeling of fullness after eating, plays a key role in managing food intake. Psyllium expands in the stomach after absorbing water, which may help promote a feeling of fullness and reduce the likelihood of overeating. This physical effect is part of what makes psyllium a popular tool for those working to maintain or reduce body weight through mindful eating habits.

By supporting appetite control and slowing the rate at which food leaves the stomach, psyllium may help individuals adhere to structured meal plans more comfortably. Its use is particularly common among those aiming to establish sustainable, long-term weight maintenance practices.

Supports the Gut Microbiome and Digestive Environment

Beyond its mechanical effects, psyllium also serves a valuable prebiotic function. Although not fermentable in the same way as other fibers, psyllium has been shown to support the growth of beneficial bacteria in the gut. A balanced and diverse microbiome is associated with better digestion, improved nutrient absorption, and greater immune support.

Psyllium may be particularly beneficial following disruptions to the gut environment, such as after a course of antibiotics or during periods of dietary inconsistency. It can also be helpful for individuals seeking to nurture their microbiome with a non-irritating, food-compatible fiber source.

Customer-Reported Psyllium Fiber Benefits

Psyllium fiber has quietly become a staple in the lives of those seeking a more balanced, lighter, and smoother digestive experience. With an average customer rating of 4.6 out of 5 across thousands of verified reviews, it is consistently praised for delivering comfort, regularity, and an overall sense of digestive ease. Users speak of psyllium not as a quick remedy, but as a dependable daily companion that helps restore a feeling of normalcy in the gut. Whether taken in capsule form or mixed into drinks, its presence is often subtle but impactful, helping people feel more "cleaned out," less bloated, and more in tune with their body's natural rhythm.

The reviews are filled with gratitude for how seamlessly psyllium fits into a busy lifestyle. Unlike harsher products that disrupt daily schedules or come with side effects, psyllium is appreciated for working gently, predictably, and without drama. For many, the shift is not just physical but emotional. Users describe feeling lighter, more energized, and even relieved after struggling with digestion for months or years. While its most obvious benefit is promoting regularity, reviewers often discover additional changes: reduced bloating, better control over cravings, improved comfort after meals, and a newfound sense of digestive confidence.

Use Case Patterns Observed

Many users turn to psyllium during periods of dietary transition, physical discomfort, or digestive frustration. Some begin using it after experiencing bloating that persists despite eating "healthy" or following a fitness routine. Others are advised by their doctor, nutritionist, or even a family member to start supplementing psyllium husk to improve digestion, support cholesterol balance, or simply get things moving more regularly.

There is a clear trend of users who are proactive about their health. These are people making lifestyle changes, cutting back on processed foods, increasing their vegetable intake, or trying to rebalance after years of fast-paced eating habits. Psyllium often becomes the missing piece that helps them feel the results of those changes. It is also popular among those managing fiber intake while on restrictive diets, recovering from digestive sluggishness, or trying to prevent the buildup of discomfort and bloating.

Capsules are frequently chosen for their convenience, especially among those who dislike the texture of powders. Others prefer powders for the ability to mix with cold water or add to their routine like a supplement ritual. Both forms are embraced as part of a broader move toward sustainable digestive wellness.

Feedback Insights

Across the reviews, a few consistent themes rise to the surface, relief, reliability, and a deep sense of bodily ease. Many users express surprise at how quickly they noticed improvements. One reviewer shared that although they were not expecting instant results, psyllium made a noticeable difference by the second day. Others echo the feeling of being "cleaned out" but without the harshness they had come to expect from other products.

The emotional tone is clear. Words like "gentle," "smooth," and "natural" are common. People often contrast psyllium with other fiber or detox products that caused cramps, urgency, or forced them to plan their day around the nearest bathroom. With psyllium, the experience is more subtle and controlled. Users say it works "just like it should" or "quietly in the background," allowing them to go about their day with confidence.

For those who had lived with prolonged digestive discomfort, the change feels profound. Several reviewers reflect on the feeling of finally "feeling normal" again, and how their body seemed to find its rhythm with psyllium. Some even mention it as a turning point in their wellness journey, calling it a "game changer" or saying they "wish they had started ten years ago."

The benefits go beyond the bathroom. Reviewers frequently note less bloating, more consistent appetite, and an easier time sticking with healthy eating. A few describe feeling "lighter and more energized," while others report better mornings, more comfort after meals, and a greater sense of daily well-being.

For those with specific health concerns like cholesterol management or blood sugar balance, psyllium is often described as a simple, natural way to add another layer of support, especially when diet and exercise alone were not delivering the full results they hoped for.

What stands out most is how often people describe psyllium as something they now "can't live without." Whether for digestive ease, weight control, or general health maintenance, this humble supplement has quietly earned a place in the lives of those seeking lasting, natural support.

Most Reported Benefits from Review Analysis

To better understand how Psyllium Fiber performs in real-world use, we analyzed thousands of verified customer reviews from people who use it daily to support their health. The following summary reflects the benefits most frequently mentioned by users who rated the product highly and described a positive experience. While everyone's body responds differently, repeated patterns in reviews offer valuable insight into how this supplement is most often used and appreciated.

With an overall rating of 4.6 out of 5, Psyllium Fiber is widely recognized as one of the most effective and accessible tools for promoting digestive comfort and regularity. Nearly half of all benefit-related comments highlight its role in relieving constipation and encouraging smooth, predictable bowel movements. Others describe it as a powerful aid in reducing bloating, improving gut comfort, managing appetite, and even supporting heart health when used consistently.

Below is a breakdown of the top five reported benefits based on this review analysis:

Benefit	%	Explanation
Regularity and Constipation Relief	50%	The most common benefit mentioned by users is improved bowel regularity. Many describe smoother, easier digestion, less straining, and a renewed sense of comfort and rhythm in their daily routine.

Benefit	%	Explanation
Digestive Health and Gut Function	30%	Reviewers frequently report feeling less bloated and more balanced. Psyllium appears to support overall digestive ease and helps create a more stable gut environment.
Appetite Control and Satiety	10%	Some users note feeling fuller for longer after taking psyllium. This helps reduce cravings between meals and supports more mindful eating habits.
Weight Management Support	5%	A smaller group of users mention weight-related improvements, often linked to reduced overeating and better digestion. It is most commonly praised as part of a larger wellness or dietary shift.
Cholesterol Balance	5%	A modest but meaningful number of users describe improved cholesterol numbers or healthier lipid profiles, particularly when psyllium is used alongside other heart-healthy habits.

How to Use This Guide

If you're considering Psyllium Fiber for a specific wellness goal, this summary can help you understand what benefits others have most consistently reported. For example, if digestive irregularity is your main concern, you may find it reassuring that regularity and constipation relief make up nearly half of all positive feedback. Likewise, if you're focused on supporting gut comfort or appetite control, those categories are also commonly highlighted by satisfied users.

These percentages do not guarantee individual results, but they do provide a useful snapshot of how Psyllium Fiber is experienced by people with a wide range of needs and lifestyles. Many users report feeling noticeable changes within a few days to a few weeks, especially when taken consistently with adequate hydration.

As always, it's important to listen to your body and consult with a healthcare provider when introducing new supplements. Psyllium Fiber is not a cure or treatment, but for many, it serves as a reliable, natural support for digestive health and overall wellness.

How to Use Psyllium Husk Fiber

Adding Psyllium Husk Fiber to your routine is simple, flexible, and easy to adapt to your personal lifestyle. Whether you prefer the convenience of capsules or the versatility of powder, there are several ways to incorporate this gentle, plant-based fiber into your daily rhythm.

The powdered form is one of the most popular options. It can be stirred into water, juice, or smoothies and consumed immediately. Some users enjoy it first thing in the morning, while others prefer it before meals or in the evening. Because psyllium thickens quickly once mixed with liquid, it is best to drink it promptly after preparing to ensure a smoother experience.

For those who prefer a no-mix option, capsules offer a tasteless, travel-friendly alternative. This format is especially useful for people with busy schedules, or anyone who prefers to avoid the texture of fiber drinks. Capsules can be taken with meals or between them, depending on individual needs and preferences.

Psyllium can also be incorporated into cooking. Some users blend it into baked goods such as muffins, pancakes, or homemade breads. This approach offers a creative way to increase fiber intake without making major changes to your existing diet.

Regardless of the form you choose, hydration is essential. Always take psyllium with a full glass of water and continue to drink fluids throughout the day. This helps the fiber work properly in the digestive tract and supports overall comfort.

It is generally best to start with a small amount and allow your body to adjust gradually. Begin with a lower dose for the first few days, then slowly increase to the recommended amount based on your body's needs and how you feel. Some people notice benefits within a day or two, while others may see changes over a longer period with consistent use.

Psyllium Husk Fiber works best as part of a balanced, long-term wellness routine. When used regularly and responsibly, it can be a helpful tool to support your fiber intake and contribute to a greater sense of daily well-being.

Omega 3 and Antioxidants

Omega-3 fatty acids and antioxidant nutrients are among the most respected and widely studied tools in nutritional wellness. Each plays a distinct yet complementary role in supporting the body's ability to function, adapt, and thrive under the demands of modern life. While Omega-3s help maintain a healthy inflammatory balance, antioxidants protect cells from the stress of daily living. Together, they provide a powerful foundation for sustaining vitality at every stage of life.

Omega-3s: Supporting Balance from the Inside Out

Omega-3 fatty acids, particularly EPA (eicosapentaenoic acid) and DHA (docosahexaenoic acid), are critical components of cellular membranes and play a central role in maintaining fluidity, communication, and resilience throughout the body. These essential fats help support cardiovascular function, brain performance, and the regulation of immune responses. They are especially valued for their role in helping the body manage inflammation in a natural and balanced way.

Despite their importance, Omega-3s are often lacking in modern diets, particularly those high in processed foods or low in fatty fish and plant-based sources. This makes mindful supplementation a key part of many people's long-term wellness strategy. In this chapter, we'll explore several forms of Omega-3 supplementation, including fish oil, algae oil, and fish eggs, and how individuals are incorporating them into daily routines to support physical and cognitive well-being.

Antioxidants: Nutrients That Safeguard Cellular Integrity

Where Omega-3s help regulate inflammation, antioxidant compounds help protect cells from oxidative stress, a process that occurs naturally as the body metabolizes food, manages stress, and is exposed to environmental factors like pollution and sunlight. Oxidative stress results from the accumulation of free radicals, unstable molecules that can impact cellular health over time.

Antioxidants work by neutralizing these free radicals, helping maintain the body's internal balance and supporting healthy aging. Among the most widely discussed antioxidants are Coenzyme Q10 (CoQ10), Resveratrol, and Shilajit. Each offers its own unique strengths:

CoQ10 plays a key role in cellular energy production and is especially important for tissues with high energy demands, such as the heart and muscles.

Resveratrol, a polyphenol found in grapes and berries, is known for supporting cardiovascular and mitochondrial health, and is frequently associated with healthy aging.

Shilajit, a natural mineral resin, delivers a rich array of trace minerals and fulvic acid, which help support antioxidant activity, nutrient transport, and cellular repair.

These antioxidant nutrients are often used alongside Omega-3s to help create a broader, more adaptive approach to wellness.

Synergizing Omega-3s, Antioxidants, and Foundational Therapies

In today's world, the body is constantly adapting to internal and external stress, ranging from poor diet and emotional pressure to environmental toxins and physical overexertion. Inflammation and oxidative stress often occur together under these conditions, which is why Omega-3s and antioxidants are frequently taken in combination. Omega-3 fatty acids help regulate inflammatory signaling, while antioxidants like CoQ10, Resveratrol, and Shilajit defend cells from oxidative damage, promoting energy, mental clarity, and long-term cellular integrity.

But their benefits are not limited to isolated effects. When used together, these compounds offer layered support, strengthening the cardiovascular system, protecting brain and nerve tissue, promoting smoother skin, and supporting recovery from physical or metabolic stress. This synergy is why many individuals include both Omega-3s and antioxidant-rich nutrients in their supplement routines.

These benefits are amplified further when paired with foundational natural therapies such as herbs, medicinal mushrooms, and nutrient-rich animal organ supplements. For example, herbs like turmeric, ginger, and licorice help prime the digestive system and reduce systemic inflammation, improving the absorption and utilization of antioxidants. Mushrooms such as Reishi and Lion's Mane contribute additional immune-modulating and neuroprotective effects, reinforcing the actions of Omega-3s and Resveratrol.

Organ supplements from sources like liver and heart provide vital cofactors, such as B vitamins, iron, and naturally occurring CoQ10, that support mitochondrial function, hormonal balance, and tissue repair. These building blocks enhance the body's capacity to respond to stress, recover from fatigue, and sustain energy and resilience over time.

Together, these therapies form an integrative wellness strategy. Rather than targeting a single symptom or concern, they help establish whole-body vitality. By supporting foundational systems, including energy metabolism, immune balance, and cellular repair, this combined approach equips your body to thrive under pressure and recover more efficiently, all while promoting long-term wellness and clarity.

Whether your focus is on boosting energy, protecting the heart and brain, reducing inflammation, or simply aging well, pairing Omega-3s and antioxidants with foundational therapies offers a powerful and practical way to support long-term health. This holistic approach fosters not just improvement, but sustained vitality and resilience through every stage of life.

Omega-3s for Lifelong Health

Omega-3 fatty acids are among the most vital nutrients for supporting long-term health, energy, and resilience. These essential fats play an integral role in maintaining the structure and function of every cell in the body. They support cardiovascular balance, cognitive performance, immune function, mood, and metabolic health. Unlike some nutrients that the body can produce on its own, Omega-3s must be consumed through food or supplementation, making them foundational to any well-rounded wellness strategy.

Omega-3s belong to a group of polyunsaturated fats that are categorized into three primary forms:

EPA (Eicosapentaenoic Acid): Known for helping support the body's natural inflammatory response, EPA is particularly associated with cardiovascular, immune, and mood-related functions.

DHA (Docosahexaenoic Acid): A primary structural component of the brain, eyes, and nervous system, DHA is essential for clear thinking, memory, and communication between cells.

ALA (Alpha-Linolenic Acid): Found in plant-based sources like flaxseeds, chia seeds, and walnuts, ALA is a precursor to EPA and DHA. However, the body's ability to convert ALA is limited, which is why direct sources of EPA and DHA are typically emphasized for optimal benefit.

These nutrients are naturally present in fatty fish such as salmon, mackerel, sardines, and anchovies, and to a lesser extent in certain algae and plant foods. However, for many individuals, obtaining enough Omega-3s from food alone can be a challenge, especially in the context of modern diets.

Why the Omega Balance Matters

The conversation around Omega-3s is incomplete without considering their dietary counterpart: Omega-6 fatty acids. Both Omega-3 and Omega-6 fats are essential for the body and play important roles in immune function, hormone signaling, and cellular structure. However, they must exist in balance to function optimally.

Historically, traditional human diets featured a balanced intake of Omega-6 to Omega-3, roughly 2:1 or 3:1. Today, in many industrialized countries, that ratio has shifted dramatically, often exceeding 10:1 or even 20:1, in favor of Omega-6. This imbalance is largely due to the increased consumption of vegetable oils (such as soybean, corn, and sunflower oil), processed foods, and packaged meals, combined with a significant reduction in Omega-3-rich foods like oily fish and seeds.

This modern dietary pattern may disrupt internal balance, especially in areas like immune regulation, tissue repair, and cardiovascular support. Omega-6 fats are not inherently harmful, but when consumed in disproportionate quantities, they may overwhelm the regulatory effects of Omega-3s.

Rebalancing Through Food and Supplementation

Addressing this imbalance doesn't require eliminating Omega-6 fats altogether. Instead, the focus is on increasing the intake of Omega-3s to restore a healthier ratio. For some people, that means eating fatty fish twice a week and using oils like olive or avocado in place of processed seed oils. For others, particularly those with dietary restrictions or limited access to fresh seafood, high-quality Omega-3 supplements can provide a convenient and reliable solution.

Supplement forms such as fish oil, algae oil, and fish egg extract offer concentrated sources of EPA and DHA, making it easier to meet daily needs. These supplements are often used by individuals seeking to support their heart, brain, joints, or overall vitality through consistent and measurable nutritional support.

Science-Informed Omega-3 Benefits

Omega-3 fatty acids are some of the most extensively studied nutrients in the field of nutritional science. As essential fats that the body cannot produce on its own, they must be obtained through diet or supplementation to support a wide range of physiological processes. Omega-3s play important roles in cellular structure, immune signaling, metabolic regulation, and neurological communication. The most well-known Omega-3s, EPA (eicosapentaenoic acid) and DHA (docosahexaenoic acid), are primarily found in fatty fish and marine oils, while ALA (alpha-linolenic acid), a plant-based Omega-3, is present in flaxseeds, chia seeds, and walnuts.

Below is a detailed overview of the primary health-supporting functions of Omega-3s, based on current research and expert consensus.

Helps Support a Balanced Inflammatory Response and Joint Mobility

Omega-3 fatty acids, particularly EPA, are involved in the regulation of the body's inflammatory signaling pathways. In response to internal or external stress, the immune system produces signaling molecules that can either promote or resolve inflammation. Omega-3s are associated with the production of compounds that help shift the body toward resolution rather than prolonged inflammatory activity.

This function is especially relevant for individuals experiencing occasional joint stiffness or discomfort. Research indicates that consistent Omega-3 intake may support smoother joint function and greater ease of movement by promoting a healthier inflammatory environment within tissues.

Promotes Cardiovascular Function and Lipid Balance

Cardiovascular health is one of the most established areas of Omega-3 research. EPA and DHA contribute to multiple aspects of heart function, including supporting healthy triglyceride levels, vascular flexibility, and circulatory flow. Omega-3s may also assist in maintaining blood vessel integrity and reducing oxidative stress within the cardiovascular system.

Numerous studies suggest that individuals with higher Omega-3 intake tend to have more favorable lipid profiles and may experience better overall cardiovascular efficiency. These benefits are most pronounced when Omega-3s are included as part of a heart-conscious lifestyle that also incorporates whole foods, physical activity, and stress management.

Supports Cognitive Clarity and Brain Cell Communication

DHA is a critical structural component of brain tissue and contributes to the formation and maintenance of neuronal membranes. It plays a vital role in the transmission of signals between nerve cells and supports brain plasticity, which is essential for memory, focus, and learning.

Omega-3s are frequently explored for their potential role in maintaining cognitive sharpness, particularly in aging populations. They are also of interest for individuals seeking support with attention, mental clarity, and overall brain vitality. While research is ongoing, consistent Omega-3 intake is associated with supporting long-term cognitive function and neurological resilience.

Encourages Emotional Stability and Neurochemical Balance

EPA has been studied for its role in modulating neurotransmitter activity, particularly in pathways involving serotonin and dopamine, two chemicals closely linked to mood regulation. A number of observational and clinical studies suggest a correlation between higher Omega-3 intake and emotional well-being, including more balanced responses to stress and improved mood resilience.

Omega-3s are often included in comprehensive wellness plans aimed at supporting emotional balance, especially during times of transition, low energy, or increased mental demand. Their influence on neurochemical balance makes them a promising area of study in the field of mental wellness.

Assists in Metabolic Regulation and Energy Efficiency

Omega-3s have been shown to influence how the body processes and stores energy. They are involved in improving cellular sensitivity to insulin and in promoting the oxidation of fatty acids, meaning they help the body use fat more efficiently as a fuel source. These properties are especially relevant for those working toward balanced energy levels and metabolic stability.

When combined with a healthy diet and regular activity, Omega-3 intake may support a more efficient metabolic state. This includes better energy regulation, reduced post-meal fatigue, and more stable appetite patterns.

Contributes to Eye Health and Visual Function

DHA is also a major structural fat in the retina, the light-sensitive tissue at the back of the eye. Adequate DHA levels support the integrity of retinal cells and may help maintain normal visual processing. In addition, Omega-3s are being studied for their role in tear production and ocular surface hydration, which can be particularly beneficial for individuals who experience occasional dry eyes or discomfort related to screen exposure.

Omega-3s may be helpful for those seeking to support long-term visual function and overall eye comfort, especially in modern environments that place heavy demands on visual focus.

Sources of Omega-3

Understanding the different sources of Omega-3s can help you choose the most effective and sustainable option for your personal needs. While EPA and DHA are the most bioactive forms of Omega-3s in the body, the way they are delivered, whether through food or supplements, can affect absorption, sustainability, and suitability for different dietary preferences. In this section, we explore the most widely used Omega-3 sources and also introduce alternatives for those with dietary restrictions or sensitivities.

Fish Eggs: A Whole-Food Source of EPA and DHA

Fish eggs, also known as roe, are a nutrient-dense and naturally balanced source of Omega-3 fatty acids. They offer both EPA and DHA in a highly bioavailable form, along with additional nutrients such as vitamin A, vitamin D, protein, and antioxidant compounds.

As a whole-food option, fish eggs provide a synergistic blend of nutrients that many individuals find supportive for overall wellness, particularly for heart, brain, and immune function.

Traditionally consumed as part of ancestral diets, fish eggs are now also available in supplement form. Freeze-dried fish egg capsules offer a convenient way to access their benefits without preparation, while preserving their nutrient profile. This makes them an attractive option for those who prefer food-based supplementation or are seeking an alternative to processed oils.

Fish Oil: Widely Researched and Concentrated

Fish oil remains one of the most popular Omega-3 supplements due to its high concentration of EPA and DHA. It has been the focus of extensive research for its role in supporting cardiovascular function, brain performance, joint comfort, and more. Fish oil is typically derived from cold-water fish such as anchovies, sardines, or mackerel, and is available in both liquid and capsule forms.

While fish oil is effective for many people, some users report experiencing a fishy aftertaste or digestive discomfort. Newer formulations, including enteric-coated capsules and triglyceride-bound oils, have helped improve tolerance and absorption. For individuals without dietary restrictions, fish oil offers a well-supported and accessible path to Omega-3 intake.

Algae Oil: A Plant-Based Source of EPA and DHA

Algae oil provides a clean, sustainable, and plant-based alternative to fish-derived Omega-3s. It is one of the only non-animal sources that delivers EPA and DHA directly, without requiring conversion from other forms. Algae oil is especially valuable for vegetarians, vegans, or individuals with seafood allergies, and is often cultivated in controlled environments to ensure purity and environmental responsibility.

Unlike plant sources like flax or chia, which primarily provide ALA, algae oil supplies the active forms of Omega-3s in a format that the body can absorb and utilize efficiently. As awareness of sustainability and dietary diversity grows, algae oil has become a trusted option for those seeking both efficacy and ethical alignment in their supplements.

Flaxseed Oil: A Plant-Based Source with Limited Conversion

Flaxseed oil is a rich source of alpha-linolenic acid (ALA), the plant-based Omega-3 precursor. It is commonly used by individuals following plant-based or allergy-conscious diets. While ALA is essential and beneficial, the body must convert it into EPA and DHA to produce the full spectrum of Omega-3 effects. This conversion is typically limited, with estimates suggesting that only a small percentage of ALA transforms into its more active forms.

Because of this limitation, flaxseed oil may be best viewed as a supportive addition rather than a standalone solution for those aiming to optimize EPA and DHA levels. Still, it remains a valuable nutritional tool, especially when used alongside other supportive dietary practices.

Beef Brain: A Nutrient-Dense Animal Source

Beef brain is a lesser-known but meaningful source of DHA, especially for those following a whole-food, nutrient-dense approach to health. As a traditional food valued in many ancestral diets, beef brain offers not only Omega-3s but also phospholipids, cholesterol, and other nutrients that support brain and nerve tissue structure.

Although not as widely available as fish oil or algae oil, beef brain is typically offered in freeze-dried capsule form and may appeal to those interested in organ-based supplementation. For readers seeking a deeper exploration of this unique source, including how it fits into broader health strategies. More information is available in the *Animal Organ Therapy* volume of this series.

Choosing the Right Omega-3 Source

Each Omega-3 source offers its own advantages, whether it's the convenience and extensive research behind fish oil, the sustainability of algae oil, the traditional nutrient density of fish eggs, or the alternative approaches offered by flaxseed oil and beef brain. Your choice may depend on personal preferences, dietary restrictions, ethical values, or how your body responds to different formats.

Importantly, for individuals who are allergic to or sensitive to marine-based sources such as fish or algae, there are still viable options. Flaxseed oil offers a plant-based way to increase Omega-3 intake, while beef brain provides a nutrient-rich animal-based alternative with natural DHA. Both options allow individuals with sensitivities to continue supporting their Omega-3 needs through non-marine sources.

By understanding the strengths and considerations of each source, you can make informed decisions that align with your wellness goals. No matter which path you take, maintaining consistent Omega-3 intake is a foundational step toward long-term health, cellular balance, and overall vitality.

Omega-3 for Vegetarians: Why Algae Oil Outshines Flax

For individuals following a vegetarian or vegan lifestyle, getting enough Omega-3 fatty acids can feel challenging, especially when most well-known sources include fish oil or fish-derived supplements. The good news is that effective, plant-based options do exist, and understanding the differences between them is key to choosing the right solution for your body and values.

Flaxseeds, chia seeds, hemp seeds, and walnuts are some of the most popular plant-based sources of Omega-3s. These foods provide alpha-linolenic acid (ALA), the essential fatty acid that serves as a precursor to EPA and DHA, the two forms of Omega-3 that the body uses most efficiently. While ALA is beneficial in its own right, the human body converts it to EPA and DHA at a very limited rate. In many people, only a small percentage of ALA is converted, meaning that even a generous intake of these plant foods may not provide sufficient levels of active Omega-3s.

This is where algae oil becomes a standout solution. Algae are the original source of DHA and EPA in the marine food chain, and fish accumulate these fatty acids by consuming algae. By going straight to the source, algae oil delivers the same beneficial compounds found in fish, but in a completely plant-based and sustainable format. It bypasses the need for conversion, offering direct access to DHA and EPA in a form the body can absorb and utilize effectively.

Algae oil is especially well-suited for individuals who follow a vegetarian or vegan lifestyle and want an alternative to fish-based sources of Omega-3s. It's also a valuable option for those with seafood allergies or sensitivities, or for anyone who finds traditional fish oil unpleasant due to the fishy aftertaste or so-called "fish burps." In addition, algae oil appeals to environmentally conscious consumers who prioritize sustainability and prefer plant-based, ocean-friendly sources of nutrition.

In addition to being a clean and effective source of Omega-3s, algae oil is produced in controlled environments, minimizing exposure to ocean-based contaminants and preserving marine ecosystems. It's a forward-thinking solution that supports both personal health and planetary health.

By choosing algae oil, individuals who avoid animal products can confidently meet their Omega-3 needs without compromising on efficacy or ethics. Whether you're following a plant-based lifestyle for health, environmental, or personal reasons, this option ensures you don't have to miss out on the well-documented benefits of these vital fatty acids.

Application of Omega-3 Supplements

Adding Omega-3 supplements to your daily wellness routine is one of the simplest ways to support foundational health. These essential fats, most notably EPA (eicosapentaenoic acid) and DHA (docosahexaenoic acid), play important roles in heart function, brain health, inflammation balance, and cellular integrity. Supplementing with Omega-3s can help bridge nutritional gaps in modern diets that often lack sufficient levels of these beneficial fatty acids.

Omega-3 supplements are available in a variety of forms, including fish oil, algae oil, and fish egg capsules. Each offers its own advantages. Fish oil is the most widely used and researched option, while fish eggs provide a nutrient-dense, whole-food alternative with additional fat-soluble vitamins. Algae oil is an excellent plant-based source of DHA, offering a clean and sustainable choice for vegetarians, vegans, or anyone with fish sensitivities.

For general health support, a consistent daily dose of Omega-3s may help promote cardiovascular resilience, cognitive clarity, and overall vitality. Since Omega-3 fatty acids are best absorbed with dietary fat, it is recommended to take them with meals, often breakfast or lunch, for optimal absorption and to help establish a lasting routine.

Individuals focusing on specific wellness goals may tailor their intake further. For example, those looking to support cardiovascular health, balance blood lipids, or address inflammation may benefit from higher doses of EPA and DHA. Likewise, individuals interested in cognitive performance may choose to prioritize DHA-rich sources for long-term brain support. It's important to follow the guidelines provided on the supplement label and consult a healthcare provider for personalized recommendations, especially if managing a specific health condition.

Algae oil is particularly valuable for those following a plant-based diet or seeking a more sustainable source of Omega-3s. Because algae are the original producers of EPA and DHA in the marine food chain, this direct source bypasses fish entirely while still delivering bioavailable essential fats.

When selecting an Omega-3 supplement, quality matters. Look for products that are third-party tested for purity and potency, especially to ensure they are free from heavy metals and oxidation. Enteric-coated capsules or those with added natural flavors can help minimize common side effects, such as fishy burps or aftertaste.

Whether your goal is to support heart rhythm, mental clarity, skin hydration, joint comfort, or overall energy, Omega-3 supplementation can be a powerful and versatile addition to your health regimen. With consistent use and the right form for your body and lifestyle, these essential fats offer lasting support for long-term well-being.

Fish Oil

Customer-Reported Fish Oil Benefits

Fish oil is by far the most widely used Omega-3 supplement in the world, and for good reasons. With thousands of reviews and a long-standing reputation in both natural health and clinical research, fish oil has earned its place as a trusted tool for supporting heart health, joint mobility, mental clarity, mood stability, and more. Across a wide spectrum of users, from busy professionals to aging adults and even athletes, fish oil is praised not just for what it offers on paper, but for how it helps people feel in daily life. Many reviewers describe meaningful shifts in energy, mental focus, mood, and physical comfort that they attribute to consistent use of a high-quality fish oil supplement.

With an impressive average rating of 4.6 out of 5, fish oil continues to be a foundational choice for those seeking long-term health and balance. Whether taken for cardiovascular support, brain performance, or simply to maintain overall well-being, users frequently express a sense of confidence that they are investing in something that truly makes a difference.

Use Case Patterns Observed

Many users turn to fish oil after learning about its wide-ranging benefits but often arrive with very specific goals in mind. One of the most common motivations is support for joint comfort and inflammation, particularly among those dealing with stiffness, pain, or reduced mobility. Others begin using fish oil to support healthy cholesterol or triglyceride levels, often as part of a broader wellness plan or under the guidance of a healthcare provider.

A second group includes individuals who report concerns related to mood swings, focus, or mental fatigue. Several reviewers describe adding fish oil during periods of stress, burnout, or emotional imbalance, and notice a surprising shift in clarity, patience, or emotional steadiness.

Another clear pattern emerges around energy and recovery, especially among those with demanding lifestyles or physically active routines. Some users say they began taking fish oil for general wellness but soon noticed faster recovery from workouts, improved sleep quality, and greater resilience throughout the day.

Fish oil is also widely chosen by people seeking long-term preventative support. These users may not have an immediate symptom to address but are motivated by a desire to nourish their heart, brain, and immune system through consistent, research-backed supplementation. In all cases, fish oil is seen as a powerful foundational tool, something that integrates naturally into their routine while quietly enhancing key areas of health.

Feedback Insights

Across reviews, one of the strongest emotional themes is surprise as many users did not expect fish oil to make such a noticeable difference. Some mention feeling better "from the inside out," reporting improved skin glow, greater mental sharpness, and fewer aches and pains in the background of daily life. Several reviewers describe how they didn't fully realize how out of balance they felt until the improvements started showing up, like sleeping through the night without pain, feeling calmer in stressful moments, or waking up without the usual stiffness in their joints.

Others express gratitude for the emotional steadiness and sense of well-being they feel after adding fish oil. Reviewers frequently describe subtle but consistent improvements in mood, mental focus, and emotional resilience. Many say it helps them feel "more themselves," especially during times of stress or hormonal fluctuation.

Digestive comfort is another commonly mentioned benefit. Many appreciate that certain brands, especially those in triglyceride form with added lemon flavoring, avoid the dreaded "fishy burps" or aftertaste. Users who had previously avoided fish oil due to digestive sensitivity often note that switching to a high-purity, well-formulated product changed their entire experience, making it easier to stick with the supplement long-term.

Finally, there is a recurring tone of commitment. Once users find a fish oil that works for them, they tend to stay loyal. Many reviewers state that they will continue taking it "for life" and recommend it to friends, family members, or even their pets. For them, fish oil is not just another supplement; it becomes part of a sustainable, empowering wellness routine.

Most Reported Benefits from Review Analysis

Fish oil continues to stand out as one of the most widely used and highly rated nutritional supplements, with thousands of users reporting measurable improvements in both how they feel and function. With an average satisfaction rating of 4.6 out of 5, fish oil earns praise across a broad spectrum of wellness goals, from supporting heart and brain health to improving skin clarity and easing joint discomfort.

To better understand how fish oil is experienced in the real world, we conducted an in-depth analysis of verified customer reviews. This analysis focused on identifying the benefits most frequently mentioned by users who reported positive outcomes. While individual results will always vary, the frequency of these reported benefits offers a helpful window into the most common areas where people feel fish oil is making a difference in their health.

For example, when 50% of reviewers describe noticeable improvements in areas tied to omega support, such as inflammation, circulation, or overall energy, that points to a consistent pattern across a wide range of individuals. Similarly, strong feedback around heart, brain, skin, and joint health gives us a clearer picture of how fish oil is being used and why so many choose to keep it in their daily routine.

Below is a summary table of fish oil's most frequently reported benefits:

Benefit	%	Explanation
Omega Support	50%	Many users report a general sense of improved well-being tied to reduced inflammation, better energy, and more balanced health. Omega-3s are credited with helping users feel sharper, calmer, and more resilient overall.
Heart Health	16%	A significant number of reviewers mention improvements in blood pressure, cholesterol, and circulation, often noting a greater sense of cardiovascular confidence.
Brain Health	13%	Enhanced cognitive clarity, focus, and mental sharpness are frequently mentioned, especially by those managing stress, mental fatigue, or aging-related concerns.
Skin Health	13%	Several users highlight clearer, more hydrated skin and a noticeable glow or reduction in dryness, especially in colder climates or after prolonged deficiency.

Benefit	%	Explanation
Joint Support	9%	Users experiencing stiffness or joint discomfort often note improved flexibility, greater ease of movement, and less daily tension after consistent use.

How to Use This Table

If you are exploring fish oil as part of your health regimen, this table offers a helpful starting point. Each percentage reflects how often a particular benefit was mentioned among users who shared a positive experience, not a guarantee, but a pattern based on widespread use.

If your main concern is inflammation or cardiovascular health, you may be especially encouraged by the large number of reviewers who report benefits in those areas. Likewise, if you're seeking support for clearer thinking, smoother skin, or joint mobility, these data-backed trends offer valuable insight into what others have found helpful.

Keep in mind that many users report multiple benefits over time, and that consistency plays a key role. Whether you are taking fish oil for a specific reason or simply as a daily foundational support, this supplement remains one of the most frequently praised tools for whole-body health and long-term vitality.

Algae Oil

Customer-Reported Algae Oil Benefits

Algae oil has emerged as the most trusted plant-based source of omega-3 fatty acids, offering a sustainable and effective alternative for those who avoid fish or seek cleaner, more eco-conscious supplements. With an impressive average rating of 4.7 out of 5, this vegan-friendly option consistently receives praise for its purity, gentleness on digestion, and surprisingly powerful impact on energy, mood, eye comfort, and overall wellness. Many users turn to algae oil not just because it fits their lifestyle, but because they've seen and felt the difference it makes. Whether for joint comfort, mental clarity, dry eye relief, or simply avoiding fishy aftertastes, algae oil has earned a loyal following across a diverse range of users.

Algae oil is especially appreciated by vegetarians, vegans, and those with seafood allergies or sensitivities. It is often discovered during a transition away from fish-based products, either for health, environmental, or ethical reasons. And while the motivation may begin with avoiding fish, many reviewers stay with algae oil because of the benefits they begin to notice over time, from sharper thinking to smoother skin. For many, it becomes more than a substitute; it becomes a long-term wellness solution in its own right.

Use Case Patterns Observed

Algae oil is most often introduced into a person's routine out of necessity, whether due to dietary preferences, allergies, or poor experiences with fish oil. Some users describe having tried multiple fish oil brands, only to be plagued by acid reflux, unpleasant burps, or lingering fishy taste. Others report digestive sensitivity, ethical concerns about marine life, or a growing awareness of the environmental cost of traditional omega sourcing.

Many users discover algae oil during a health journey, often prompted by recommendations from doctors, eye care specialists, or functional medicine practitioners. It is commonly used for managing dryness (especially dry eye syndrome), supporting cognitive focus and memory, regulating mood, and maintaining cardiovascular balance. A number of reviewers also turn to algae oil to complement treatments for inflammatory conditions or as a natural aid during periods of physical or emotional stress.

Parents, busy professionals, aging adults, and individuals managing mood or eye issues frequently report that algae oil becomes a daily essential. Some reviewers also highlight its use during pregnancy, with one user pointing out its role in child development through DHA support, especially when meat or fish intake is limited.

Feedback Insights

The tone of customer feedback for algae oil is overwhelmingly positive, with many reviewers expressing relief, gratitude, and even surprise at how much better they felt after making the switch. Words like "gentle," "clean," "calm," "focused," and "relieved" are common. One user, who switched due to a fish allergy, said they "felt smarter" and that their memory noticeably improved. Others described finally finding a supplement they could take without discomfort: "No fish burps, no acid reflux, just clarity and calm."

A recurring theme is the emotional comfort users feel from knowing they are getting high-quality omega-3s without compromising their ethics or harming the environment. One reviewer celebrated that algae oil is "a supplement with the ocean in mind," while another called it "the superior omega-3" because it skips the fish entirely and leaves no aftertaste. Several mentioned feeling empowered that their choice was both effective and aligned with their values.

Many also speak about the tangible physical improvements they noticed, such as reduced eye dryness, better joint flexibility, and increased emotional resilience. Some described more restful sleep, steadier energy, and fewer mood swings. A user who had been suffering from hip pain for years found that after just a few weeks of algae oil, their pain had diminished significantly, only to return when they ran out. That contrast reinforced how impactful the supplement had been.

For those with sensitive systems, algae oil stood out for its tolerability. One reviewer with a history of gastric bypass surgery noted that even high doses caused no issues, and another shared that they switched from multiple failed fish oil attempts due to stomach upset and finally found algae oil to be "the one that works."

In the end, what shines through most in the feedback is not just satisfaction, but transformation. Algae oil isn't just a substitute for fish oil, it is a trusted daily ally that supports health with purity, purpose, and peace of mind.

Most Reported Benefits from Review Analysis

Algae oil has quickly become a trusted solution for individuals seeking a clean, plant-based source of omega-3s. With an exceptional average customer rating of 4.7 out of 5, this supplement is praised for delivering real-world results across several key areas of wellness. Users consistently report noticeable improvements in cardiovascular function, cognitive clarity, cholesterol balance, and overall well-being.

To better understand what people are experiencing, we analyzed thousands of verified reviews and identified the most frequently mentioned benefits. The percentages shown below reflect how often each benefit appears among users with positive experiences. While individual results vary, a higher percentage suggests a consistent pattern of effectiveness across a broad range of users.

For instance, 84 percent of reviewers specifically referenced improvements related to omega-3 support. This includes better heart and brain function, reduced inflammation, and greater overall wellness. If these are your goals, algae oil may be especially worth considering.

Algae Oil's Top Benefits Reported by Customers

Benefit	%	Explanation
Omega support	84%	Most users report improved heart and brain function, reduced inflammation, and overall vitality from consistent omega-3 intake.
Brain health	6%	Many users highlight enhanced mental clarity, focus, and cognitive support.
Heart health	6%	Reviewers mention improvements in cardiovascular wellness, including better circulation and blood pressure balance.
Cholesterol management	3%	Some users report more stable lipid profiles and improved cholesterol numbers.
Memory support	1%	A smaller group shares experiences of sharper recall and reduced mental fog.

How to Use This Table

This summary offers a snapshot of what people commonly experience when using algae oil as part of their wellness routine. These percentages are not meant to predict individual outcomes, but they do highlight areas where the supplement has gained consistent praise from users.

If you are looking to support your cardiovascular system, reduce inflammation, or improve cognitive function, particularly through a non-fish-based supplement, algae oil may be a good fit. With a high satisfaction rating and strong user-reported benefits, it has proven to be both effective and well tolerated by a wide range of individuals.

Many reviewers also note that benefits become more noticeable with consistent use over time. As with any supplement, consider your unique needs, consult a qualified health professional if necessary, and allow a few weeks of regular intake before evaluating results.

Fish Eggs

Customer-Reported Fish Eggs Benefits

Fish eggs, or roe, are gaining attention as a premium whole-food source of omega-3s and vital fat-soluble nutrients. While not as widely used as fish oil, they have earned deep loyalty from those seeking a more ancestral and nutrient-dense approach to omega-3 supplementation. With an impressive customer rating of 4.6 out of 5, users frequently describe noticeable improvements in mental clarity, energy, fertility support, mood balance, and skin health. Many feel they are receiving a full spectrum of nourishment compared to traditional omega-3 options.

Unlike processed oils, fish eggs offer a naturally concentrated source of EPA and DHA, along with vitamins A, D, E, and K2, and essential phospholipids that support brain, eye, and reproductive function. This richness is reflected in the wide range of real-world benefits reported by users, particularly those following whole-food or carnivore diets, or those seeking hormone and fertility support.

Use Case Patterns Observed

Fish eggs are most commonly chosen by individuals seeking a more complete omega-3 supplement, especially those who want to avoid fish oil due to concerns about oxidation, digestion, or purity. They are frequently used by people who follow animal-based or nutrient-dense diets, as well as those working on fertility, mood stability, and hormonal balance.

Several reviewers specifically mention using fish eggs to complement or replace prenatal vitamins, or to support natural conception.

Others turn to fish eggs for help with brain fog, fatigue, sleep quality, and stress resilience. Many users stack fish eggs with other ancestral supplements, such as beef liver, to support comprehensive wellness.

Feedback Insights

The emotional tone of the feedback is enthusiastic and often deeply grateful. Many users express a strong sense of physical and emotional improvement after adding fish eggs to their daily routine. Reviewers report feeling "more clear-headed," "stable in mood," and "energized in the morning." Some describe these supplements as a "missing piece" in their wellness routine that finally helped them feel grounded and resilient.

Users frequently note improvements in cognitive function, such as sharper memory and reduced brain fog, especially when combining fish eggs with other organ-based supplements like beef brain. Several people share that their vision became clearer, dry eyes improved, and sleep became more restful. One user observed that her "floaters almost disappeared," while another noted a return of her menstrual cycle and improved emotional balance.

For those focused on fertility, the response is particularly heartfelt. Multiple women mention improved hormonal patterns and support during conception. One shared, "I'm in my 40s and was trying to get pregnant naturally. After using these, I'm now four months pregnant."

Even those initially skeptical about the fishy taste or smell expressed surprise at how well their bodies responded. "They smell like fish eggs, but I feel incredible," one reviewer wrote. Others humorously noted that their pets could detect the smell but emphasized the benefits far outweighed the mild odor.

Most Reported Benefits from Review Analysis

Fish eggs are a highly concentrated, whole-food source of omega-3s and fat-soluble nutrients, and their benefits are consistently praised by users seeking a premium alternative to traditional fish oil. With an overall satisfaction rating of 4.6 out of 5, many users report noticeable improvements in physical energy, mental clarity, skin health, and overall vitality. These benefits appear to reflect the bioavailability of essential fatty acids, phospholipids, and fat-soluble vitamins that are naturally abundant in roe.

To better understand what users are actually experiencing, we analyzed thousands of verified reviews, identifying the benefits most frequently mentioned by satisfied customers. While individual results always vary, the percentage breakdown below highlights which benefits show up most often in real-world experiences. A higher percentage suggests a consistent pattern of positive outcomes in that area.

For example, 37 percent of reviewers specifically mentioned a boost in energy, indicating that improved stamina and reduced fatigue are among the most widely reported benefits of taking fish eggs. Brain health and skin vitality also featured prominently, reflecting the broad-spectrum nutritional impact of this ancestral superfood.

Below is a summary table of fish eggs' top benefits as reported by customers:

Benefit	%	Explanation
Energy boost	37%	Many users report a noticeable increase in energy and stamina, with reduced fatigue and a greater sense of daily vitality.

Benefit	%	Explanation
Brain health	22%	Enhanced mental clarity, focus, and cognitive sharpness are frequently noted, especially among users combining fish eggs with other nutrient-dense supplements.
Skin health	22%	Users describe clearer, more hydrated skin with improved texture, tone, and elasticity, often citing a healthy glow and reduced dryness.
Heart health	10%	Several users report feeling more balanced and supported in cardiovascular wellness, often linking this to the natural omega-3 content.
Omega support	9%	Broad-spectrum omega-3 benefits, including support for brain, heart, joints, and hormonal balance, are commonly mentioned by those seeking whole-food alternatives to fish oil.

How to Use This Table

These percentages reflect how often each benefit was mentioned among users who had a positive experience with fish egg supplements. They are not guarantees of specific outcomes but offer a helpful window into what others have noticed most consistently. If you are exploring fish eggs for a particular health goal, such as boosting energy, improving skin, or supporting brain performance, these insights can guide your expectations and help you decide whether this whole-food omega source aligns with your needs.

It is worth noting that many users report multiple benefits at once, and results often become more noticeable with consistent use over time. As part of a nutrient-rich wellness plan, fish eggs may provide a valuable foundation for sustained energy, cognitive vitality, and overall well-being.

Antioxidants for Cellular Defense

Antioxidants are essential compounds that help defend the body against oxidative stress, an internal process that occurs when there is an imbalance between free radicals and the body's ability to neutralize them. Free radicals are unstable molecules that can accumulate from exposure to environmental toxins, processed foods, poor lifestyle habits, and even the body's natural metabolic processes. Left unchecked, these reactive compounds can damage cells, accelerate aging, and contribute to a wide range of chronic health concerns, including cardiovascular dysfunction, cognitive decline, and fatigue.

Antioxidants serve as the body's natural defense mechanism, helping to stabilize free radicals before they can cause harm. By protecting cellular structures, including DNA, proteins, and lipids, from oxidative damage, antioxidants play a central role in supporting long-term vitality, tissue repair, and resilience. They also help reduce systemic inflammation, improve immune function, and enhance energy production by supporting healthy mitochondrial activity.

In practical terms, this means antioxidants contribute to many areas of wellness that people care deeply about: maintaining heart health, preserving mental sharpness, supporting graceful aging, sustaining energy levels, and keeping the skin looking vibrant and healthy. Their benefits are particularly impactful in today's world, where environmental and emotional stressors are constantly increasing the body's oxidative burden.

Among the many antioxidant compounds available, a few stand out for their potency, unique mechanisms, and widespread use. Coenzyme Q10 (CoQ10), for example, is a vital antioxidant involved in cellular energy production and is especially beneficial for the heart and muscles. Resveratrol, a natural compound found in grapes and berries, has gained attention for its potential to support longevity, protect the brain, and enhance circulation. Shilajit, a mineral-rich resin sourced from mountainous regions, provides powerful antioxidant support along with a spectrum of bioavailable minerals that nourish the body at the cellular level.

In the following chapters, we will take a closer look at each of these antioxidant solutions, exploring how they work, what the research shows, and what customers report after consistent use. Whether you are seeking more energy, healthier aging, better heart health, or stronger mental focus, these natural compounds may offer meaningful support for your journey toward optimal well-being.

Coenzyme Q10 (CoQ10)

Coenzyme Q10, often referred to as CoQ10, is a naturally occurring compound that plays a vital role in energy production and cellular protection throughout the body. This fat-soluble antioxidant is found in every cell, with particularly high concentrations in the heart, liver, kidneys, and other energy-demanding organs. CoQ10 is essential for producing adenosine triphosphate (ATP), the molecule that powers nearly every physiological process, from muscle contraction to brain activity.

In addition to fueling cellular energy, CoQ10 serves as a key antioxidant that helps protect cells from oxidative stress, one of the primary contributors to aging and chronic disease. It neutralizes harmful free radicals that accumulate from metabolic activity, environmental exposures, and inflammatory processes. Over time, the body's natural production of CoQ10 declines, particularly with age or in individuals taking certain medications such as statins. This reduction can affect cardiovascular health, stamina, mental clarity, and overall vitality.

Supplementing with CoQ10 can help restore optimal levels, supporting mitochondrial function, protecting cells from damage, and enhancing overall well-being. Whether you are looking to support your heart, improve energy, sharpen your mind, or protect against the effects of aging, CoQ10 offers wide-ranging benefits backed by scientific research.

Science-Informed CoQ10 Benefits

Supports Heart Health and Circulation

CoQ10 plays an essential role in maintaining a healthy cardiovascular system. The heart requires a constant supply of energy to pump blood efficiently, and CoQ10 is critical to this process. It supports the function of blood vessels, helps maintain healthy blood pressure levels, and reduces oxidative stress that can damage heart tissue. Studies have shown that CoQ10 may benefit individuals with hypertension, high cholesterol, or other cardiovascular concerns. It is especially important for those taking statin medications, which are known to lower CoQ10 levels as a side effect.

Boosts Energy Production and Reduces Fatigue

By supporting mitochondrial activity, CoQ10 enhances the body's ability to generate energy. This is especially valuable for individuals experiencing persistent fatigue, low stamina, or metabolic conditions. Research indicates that CoQ10 supplementation can improve energy in people with chronic fatigue syndrome, fibromyalgia, and other conditions related to mitochondrial dysfunction. It may also support individuals seeking greater endurance or recovery from physically demanding activities.

Enhances Brain Function and Cognitive Health

Oxidative stress and inflammation are closely linked to neurodegenerative conditions such as Alzheimer's and Parkinson's disease. CoQ10 helps protect neurons by reducing oxidative damage and supporting mitochondrial energy production in the brain. Some studies suggest that it may help slow age-related cognitive decline and support mental clarity, focus, and memory. Individuals seeking to maintain brain health as they age may find CoQ10 to be a valuable addition to their wellness routine.

Protects Against Aging and Skin Damage

The skin is highly susceptible to oxidative damage caused by sun exposure, pollution, and internal metabolic stress. CoQ10 helps protect the skin by reducing free radical activity and supporting cellular repair. Research shows that it can improve skin hydration, firmness, and elasticity. In some cases, CoQ10 is also used in topical formulations to provide direct antioxidant protection and reduce visible signs of aging. Those looking to support healthy, youthful skin may benefit from both internal and topical use.

Supports Muscle Recovery and Physical Performance

CoQ10 has been shown to improve muscle function and reduce post-exercise soreness by enhancing oxygen delivery and reducing exercise-induced oxidative stress. Athletes and those recovering from physical exertion may find that CoQ10 supports faster recovery and improved endurance. Studies also suggest that it can help reduce muscle fatigue and enhance exercise performance, especially in older adults or individuals with lower baseline CoQ10 levels.

Choosing Your Source of CoQ10

As your body's natural levels of Coenzyme Q10 (CoQ10) decline with age, finding the right way to replenish this vital compound becomes increasingly important. Fortunately, there are multiple ways to support your CoQ10 needs, ranging from nutrient-rich whole foods to precisely formulated supplements. Whether your goal is heart support, energy enhancement, or general cellular protection, there's a CoQ10 source to match your health priorities and lifestyle.

Beef Heart Supplements: A Whole-Food Source of CoQ10

Beef heart supplements, previously introduced in the Foundational Therapy chapter, offer one of the most nutrient-dense and bioavailable sources of CoQ10. Derived from grass-fed bovine heart, this traditional organ supplement naturally delivers CoQ10 along with key cofactors such as amino acids, B vitamins, and trace minerals that work synergistically to support cardiovascular function and mitochondrial energy production.

As we grow older, the body's ability to maintain optimal CoQ10 levels diminishes. Beef heart supplements help bridge this nutritional gap in a form the body can easily recognize and utilize. Unlike isolated compounds, the CoQ10 found in beef heart comes embedded in a matrix of whole-food nutrients, which may enhance its absorption and biological activity. For individuals seeking a natural, food-based approach to support energy levels, heart health, and cellular vitality, beef heart provides a powerful, time-tested solution.

CoQ10-Specific Supplements: A Convenient Alternative

For those who prefer not to consume organ-based supplements or who want more control over specific dosing, CoQ10-specific supplements offer a convenient and effective alternative. Available in capsules, tablets, and softgel formats, these products make it easy to incorporate CoQ10 into your daily wellness routine.

These supplements are especially helpful for individuals with targeted health concerns such as fatigue, cardiovascular stress, or age-related decline in mitochondrial function. Whether used alongside a balanced diet or as part of a broader supplement regimen, CoQ10 capsules provide a straightforward way to support the body's energy production, antioxidant defenses, and heart function.

Ubiquinone vs. Ubiquinol: Understanding the Two Forms

When selecting a CoQ10 supplement, it's important to consider which form, ubiquinone or ubiquinol, is best suited to your needs.

Ubiquinone is the oxidized form of CoQ10 and has long been the standard choice for general supplementation. It plays a vital role in cellular energy production and is well-suited for individuals who are generally healthy and want to maintain long-term vitality.

Ubiquinol is the reduced, active form of CoQ10, and it is more easily absorbed by the body. As people age, their ability to convert ubiquinone into ubiquinol naturally decreases. For this reason, individuals over 50 or those with increased oxidative stress may benefit more from taking CoQ10 in its ubiquinol form. This enhanced bioavailability helps support energy metabolism and antioxidant protection at a time when the body may need it most.

Those with heart conditions, high levels of physical activity, or chronic fatigue may also prefer ubiquinol due to its faster absorption and greater cellular impact. While ubiquinone remains a cost-effective and valuable option, ubiquinol offers more targeted benefits for individuals with higher demands or lower conversion capacity.

Both forms are effective, and your choice should reflect your age, health goals, and current energy or cardiovascular needs. For optimal results, consider speaking with a healthcare professional to determine the best formulation and dosage for your unique situation.

Customer-Reported CoQ10 Benefits

Coenzyme Q10 (CoQ10) is widely praised by users for its ability to enhance energy, support heart function, and promote overall vitality, especially for those managing fatigue, cardiovascular concerns, or statin-related side effects. With an impressive overall customer rating of 4.6 out of 5, the real-world experiences of thousands of users offer valuable insight into how this supplement is being used and what benefits are most commonly reported. Whether taken as part of a cardiovascular health plan, for energy renewal, or in support of aging well, CoQ10 has earned a strong reputation for being both effective and well-tolerated. In the sections below, we break down how people are using CoQ10 and what they're saying about its impact on their daily lives.

Use Case Patterns Observed

CoQ10 supplementation is most commonly adopted by individuals seeking to support heart health, restore energy levels, or offset the side effects of statin medications. Many users also turn to it during periods of prolonged fatigue, after surgery, or as part of a proactive wellness plan to enhance aging resilience and cardiovascular protection. A significant number of reviewers noted starting CoQ10 due to recommendations from healthcare providers, especially following heart-related concerns, cholesterol management protocols, or persistent low energy. Others discovered it through personal research when conventional energy supplements or medications proved ineffective or came with unwanted side effects. A smaller group used CoQ10 to complement efforts around managing blood pressure, muscle weakness, or general recovery after illness or injury. The range of applications reflects CoQ10's reputation as a well-tolerated supplement for whole-body cellular energy and cardiovascular support.

Feedback Insights

The emotional tone of CoQ10 reviews is overwhelmingly positive, with users frequently expressing relief, gratitude, and even surprise at how effective the supplement turned out to be, especially when other products had fallen short. One reviewer described their experience as "finally feeling alive again," after years of waking up exhausted despite sleep, while another shared that CoQ10 helped them "crawl out of a hole" of chronic tiredness. These expressions speak to a transformation that many did not expect but welcomed with open arms.

Energy restoration was the most commonly celebrated benefit. Many users said they felt the difference within the first week, describing it as "a push through the day" instead of dragging through it. People who were once relying on excessive caffeine or struggling with daily fatigue said that CoQ10 gave them a steady, sustained form of energy that made them feel more capable and motivated.

Several reviews came from those taking statin medications who had been dealing with muscle aches, weakness, or general fatigue, issues they later learned could be linked to CoQ10 depletion. After adding this supplement to their routine, many reported marked improvements in physical comfort, joint mobility, and energy stability. Some mentioned they no longer needed extra naps, while others noted fewer nighttime cramps and better muscle recovery.

Cardiovascular health was another theme that surfaced strongly. Users shared how CoQ10 seemed to help stabilize blood pressure or improve cholesterol numbers, especially when taken consistently. Many emphasized that they were not using it in place of medical treatments, but alongside them, often at their doctor's recommendation.

A more personal yet less expected outcome reported by a number of users was better sleep. Those who struggled with irregular sleep patterns, disrupted circadian rhythms, or REM disturbances noted that after adding CoQ10, they began waking more refreshed, falling asleep faster, and experiencing deeper rest. This improved sleep then fed back into better mood and daily function, enhancing the perceived benefits even more.

Taken together, the reviews point to a supplement that users not only find effective, but one that earns their trust through tangible improvements in vitality, cardiovascular stability, and daily performance.

Most Reported Benefits from Review Analysis

Coenzyme Q10 (CoQ10) continues to earn praise from users seeking natural ways to support heart function, increase daily energy, and recover more efficiently from physical strain. With a strong average rating of 4.6 out of 5, thousands of reviewers describe feeling more energized, balanced, and physically capable after adding CoQ10 to their routines. While some discovered it through research or health professional recommendations, particularly when taking statin medications, others began taking it simply to improve fatigue or maintain cardiovascular wellness as they age.

Our analysis of these reviews highlights the specific benefits that users mention most often. The percentages reflect how frequently each benefit appeared among those reporting a positive experience. A higher percentage suggests a more common outcome, especially for those with similar wellness goals.

For example, if nearly half of all satisfied users report heart health improvements, it suggests a strong pattern of cardiovascular support, particularly in circulation, blood pressure, and stamina. These real-world patterns can help guide your expectations and give insight into how others are using CoQ10 to support their health.

Below is a summary table of CoQ10's top benefits as reported by customers:

CoQ10's Top Benefits Reported by Customers

Benefit	%	Explanation
Heart health	49%	Users frequently report improved cardiovascular function, circulation, and support while taking statins.
Energy boost	35%	Many describe feeling more energized and less sluggish, especially during busy or stressful periods.
Muscle recovery	10%	Aids in endurance and post-activity recovery, with less soreness and improved resilience.
Fatigue reduction	4%	Users note a noticeable drop in overall fatigue, with better physical and mental stamina.
Brain health	2%	Some reviewers report clearer thinking, sharper focus, and cognitive uplift.

How to Use This Table

The figures in this table are based on real customer feedback, reflecting the most frequently reported benefits among those who had a positive experience. While every individual responds differently, the higher the percentage, the more commonly that benefit was observed by others. If your goals align with one or more of these outcomes, this table can help set realistic expectations and guide your decision on whether CoQ10 may be a good fit for your needs.

These insights, coupled with its excellent customer satisfaction score, suggest that CoQ10 may be especially helpful for supporting cardiovascular wellness, increasing energy, aiding physical recovery, and promoting long-term vitality.

Application of CoQ10 Supplement

For anyone with heart disease or heart discomfort, or anyone over 50 years old, or any one with low energy, incorporating CoQ10 into your daily routine is simple and can significantly enhance your energy and heart health. For optimal absorption, take your CoQ10 supplement with a meal that contains healthy fats, such as breakfast with avocado or lunch with olive oil-based dressing. This fat helps your body absorb the fat-soluble CoQ10 more efficiently. Most adults benefit from a daily dose ranging between 100 to 200 mg, but it's best to follow the dosage recommended on the product label or by your healthcare provider based on your individual health needs.

Resveratrol: Anti-Aging Powerhouse

Resveratrol is a naturally occurring polyphenol found in the skin of red grapes, berries, and certain other plants. It has garnered considerable scientific interest for its antioxidant properties and its ability to support cellular repair, vascular health, and metabolic function. Known for its presence in red wine and certain superfoods, resveratrol plays a valuable role in helping the body manage oxidative stress, one of the key contributors to cellular aging and long-term health challenges.

As an antioxidant, resveratrol helps neutralize free radicals, unstable molecules that can cause damage to cells and tissues over time. This protective function supports a wide range of health systems, from cardiovascular integrity to metabolic regulation and neurological resilience. Resveratrol also interacts with several signaling pathways in the body, including those involved in mitochondrial function and inflammatory response, contributing to its reputation as a natural tool for supporting longevity and vitality.

Science-Informed Resveratrol Benefits

Supports Healthy Aging and Cellular Longevity

One of the most intriguing aspects of resveratrol is its interaction with sirtuins, a group of proteins involved in regulating cellular aging and stress resistance. By influencing these pathways, resveratrol helps maintain the function of mitochondria, the energy-producing structures inside cells, and supports the body's natural repair mechanisms. While aging is inevitable, supporting these systems may help individuals maintain vitality and resilience over time.

Promotes Heart and Vascular Function

Resveratrol has been studied for its effects on endothelial function, the ability of blood vessels to expand and contract effectively. Maintaining healthy endothelial activity supports optimal circulation, balanced blood pressure, and flexible arteries. Research also suggests that resveratrol may assist in managing lipid balance, particularly by supporting healthy LDL and HDL cholesterol ratios. These effects, taken together, contribute to overall cardiovascular support.

Supports Cognitive Clarity and Brain Health

Oxidative stress and chronic inflammation are known to affect brain function over time. Resveratrol's antioxidant properties help protect neural cells and support healthy cognitive aging. Preliminary research indicates that it may help promote memory retention and mental clarity, particularly when taken as part of a long-term wellness strategy. While more studies are needed, many individuals incorporate resveratrol to help maintain focus and brain resilience as they age.

Encourages Metabolic Balance and Weight Regulation

Resveratrol has been shown to support insulin sensitivity, a key factor in balanced blood sugar management. It also influences fat metabolism and may help reduce the accumulation of excess fat in the body. These actions contribute to its potential in promoting healthy metabolic function and weight maintenance, especially when paired with good nutrition and regular activity.

Contributes to Cellular Protection and Detoxification

In laboratory studies, resveratrol has demonstrated the ability to influence pathways associated with cell cycle regulation and cellular detoxification. While it is not used as a treatment, its role in supporting the body's natural defenses against cellular stress makes it a valuable component in many preventive health strategies. This may include supporting the body's natural response to DNA damage and encouraging efficient cellular turnover.

Offers Anti-Inflammatory Support

Chronic inflammation can contribute to discomfort and affect quality of life. Resveratrol has been observed to help modulate inflammatory signals in the body, offering support in maintaining joint mobility, digestive comfort, and overall systemic balance. For individuals focused on supporting long-term wellness, this property makes resveratrol a versatile addition to their daily health plan.

A Holistic Addition to a Longevity-Focused Lifestyle

Incorporating resveratrol as part of a well-rounded supplement routine offers a plant-based option for those looking to support multiple areas of wellness. Its benefits touch on heart health, cellular energy, brain clarity, and metabolic resilience, making it especially popular among individuals interested in aging gracefully and maintaining active, engaged lives.

While research into resveratrol continues, what is already known highlights its potential to promote internal balance and protect against the everyday stressors that affect cells and systems over time. Choosing a high-quality, well-sourced resveratrol supplement, and pairing it with other healthy habits, can be a proactive way to invest in long-term vitality.

Discovering Your Resveratrol Sources

Unlocking the benefits of resveratrol begins with knowing where to find this powerful compound in your daily life. Naturally, resveratrol is abundant in the skin of red grapes, making red wine a popular source for those who enjoy a glass in moderation. Berries such as blueberries, cranberries, and mulberries also pack a significant resveratrol punch, offering a delicious and nutritious way to boost your intake. Additionally, peanuts and dark chocolate are surprising yet effective sources, providing a tasty treat that contributes to your resveratrol levels. For those who prefer plant-based options, certain berries and nuts can be easily incorporated into meals and snacks, ensuring you receive the antioxidant benefits without relying on alcohol.

However, obtaining sufficient resveratrol through diet alone can be challenging, especially if you're aiming for higher therapeutic doses to maximize its health benefits. This is where resveratrol supplements come into play. Available in various forms such as capsules, tablets, and softgels, supplements offer a convenient and concentrated way to enhance your resveratrol intake. These supplements are often derived from natural sources like Japanese knotweed or red grape extract, ensuring you receive a pure and potent dose. Whether you choose to enrich your diet with resveratrol-rich foods or prefer the simplicity of supplementation, incorporating resveratrol into your wellness routine can help you harness its full potential. Always consult with a healthcare professional before starting any new supplement regimen to determine the best form and dosage for your individual health needs. By blending natural sources with thoughtful supplementation, you can effectively integrate resveratrol into your lifestyle, supporting your journey toward vibrant health and longevity.

Customer-Reported Resveratrol Benefits

Resveratrol has captivated the attention of health-conscious individuals for its association with longevity, vitality, and cellular protection. With an average satisfaction rating of 4.5 out of 5 stars, customer reviews suggest that this polyphenolic compound offers a wide range of perceived benefits across energy, skin appearance, immune resilience, cardiovascular health, and cognitive performance. While results vary, many individuals feel that resveratrol plays a subtle but consistent role in improving how they feel and function day to day. It is often described not as an immediate, dramatic change but as a gradual shift toward enhanced energy, clearer thinking, and a more youthful sense of well-being.

Use Case Patterns Observed

Most users report turning to resveratrol as part of a proactive wellness regimen rather than as a targeted intervention for a single condition. It is commonly used by individuals over 50 seeking to support graceful aging, heart function, or joint mobility. Others integrate resveratrol into their daily routine alongside NAD+ or CoQ10 as part of a broader mitochondrial or antioxidant protocol. Many reviews also reflect interest in resveratrol's role in promoting healthy blood pressure, supporting immune defenses during cold and flu season, or helping reduce joint discomfort and inflammation. A growing number of younger users report taking it for skin appearance, energy levels, and mental focus, particularly those aiming to stay ahead of aging-related changes. Whether paired with other supplements or used on its own, resveratrol is frequently adopted by those seeking to maintain vitality and prevent decline.

Feedback Insights

Reviewers often express a deep sense of appreciation for the subtle yet steady benefits they associate with resveratrol. Many describe feeling "younger," "more energetic," or "more alert," sometimes only noticing the difference when they stop taking it and fatigue or brain fog returns. One customer wrote that after running out of resveratrol, their energy dropped sharply, and once they resumed, their "previous high level" of vitality returned. Another described it as "a natural uplift" with no jitters, while a 71-year-old user credited it with helping them stay physically active and mentally engaged, noting they had resumed activities like gardening and building projects.

Cognitive clarity and memory support are commonly mentioned, with users reporting reduced brain fog and improved recall. One reviewer humorously shared that they no longer forget why they walked into a room, and another mentioned feeling sharper and more efficient throughout the day.

Many also highlight noticeable changes in skin health, including reduced wrinkles, firmer skin tone, and brighter complexion. One reviewer commented on the fading of forehead lines and sagging skin after just a few days, calling it "like a reset button for my appearance."

For joint comfort and mobility, some users report reduced knee pain and inflammation, often within a week of starting supplementation. A long-time runner nearing age 70 shared that resveratrol helped them continue running 50 miles per week with only occasional discomfort.

While a few users remain cautious about drawing direct conclusions, the overall tone is one of trust and long-term satisfaction. Words like "grateful," "rejuvenated," and "steady improvement" appear often, underscoring the sense that resveratrol, while not dramatic in effect, has become a valued part of daily health maintenance for many.

Most Reported Benefits from Review Analysis

Thousands of users turn to resveratrol in pursuit of greater vitality, resilience, and long-term wellness. Our analysis of highly rated reviews reveals consistent patterns in how people experience the benefits of this polyphenol-rich antioxidant. While each body is different, the percentages below reflect the most frequently mentioned outcomes among users who reported positive effects. A higher percentage indicates that the benefit was cited more often, offering insight into what people are most likely to notice when using resveratrol consistently.

For instance, if 30 percent of reviewers mentioned an energy boost, that suggests a meaningful portion of users felt more energized, less fatigued, and better able to engage with daily life after adding resveratrol to their routine.

Below is a summary table of Resveratrol's top benefits as reported by customers:

Benefit	%	Explanation
Energy boost	30%	Many users report a significant increase in energy, stamina, and reduced fatigue.
Heart health	28%	Supports cardiovascular function, improving circulation and maintaining healthy cholesterol levels.
Skin health	20%	Noticeable improvements in skin elasticity, hydration, and overall complexion.
Anti-aging	12%	Helps combat oxidative stress and slow down visible signs of aging.

Benefit	%	Explanation
Brain health	10%	Users experience better cognitive function, focus, and mental clarity.

How to Use This Table

This table is designed to help you understand the most commonly observed benefits based on real user experiences. It does not guarantee results, but it offers a helpful guide to what others have noticed when using resveratrol as part of their wellness regimen. If your primary interest is in energy, heart support, or skin health, these percentages suggest that you may be more likely to experience benefits in those areas. Everyone responds differently, but this data reflects patterns across thousands of individuals who felt resveratrol made a positive impact.

Whether you are exploring resveratrol for its antioxidant potential, longevity support, or everyday vitality, these insights can help you approach your supplement journey with more clarity and confidence.

Applications of Resveratrol

Incorporating resveratrol into your daily life is both simple and convenient, allowing you to harness its powerful health benefits without disrupting your busy schedule. One of the most popular and user-friendly ways to take resveratrol is through capsules. These easy-to-swallow capsules provide a precise dosage, ensuring you receive the optimal amount of this potent antioxidant with minimal effort. Whether you prefer morning or evening supplementation, resveratrol capsules can easily fit into your existing routine, whether alongside your breakfast coffee or as part of your nightly wellness regimen.

When it comes to dosage, it's essential to follow the guidelines provided on the product label or consult with a healthcare practitioner to determine the best amount for your individual needs. Most resveratrol supplements range from 150 to 500 milligrams per day, but your optimal dose may vary based on factors such as age, health status, and specific health goals. Starting with a lower dose and gradually increasing it can help your body adjust and minimize any potential side effects, such as mild digestive discomfort. Follow the directions in the product label or consult a professional as needed.

To maximize the benefits of resveratrol, consider taking your supplement with a meal that includes healthy fats, such as avocado, nuts, or olive oil. Resveratrol is fat-soluble, meaning that consuming it with fats enhances its absorption and effectiveness. Additionally, some high-quality resveratrol supplements are formulated with ingredients like piperine (derived from black pepper) to further boost bioavailability, ensuring that your body can fully utilize this powerful compound.

In addition to capsules, resveratrol is available in other convenient forms such as tablets, softgels, and even liquid extracts, allowing you to choose the method that best fits your lifestyle and preferences. Whether you prefer the simplicity of a capsule or the versatility of a liquid extract that can be added to smoothies, there's a resveratrol option to suit every need.

By thoughtfully integrating resveratrol into your daily routine through convenient supplementation, adhering to recommended dosages, and seeking professional guidance when needed, you can effectively harness the full spectrum of its health benefits. Embrace the ease and flexibility of resveratrol supplementation and take a proactive step toward enhancing your longevity, cardiovascular health, cognitive function, and overall vitality.

Shilajit: Mineral and Antioxidant

Shilajit is a rare and potent natural substance that combines the richest source of bioavailable minerals with powerful antioxidant protection. Formed over centuries from decomposed plant matter in the high-altitude regions of the Himalayas, this nutrient-dense resin has been a staple in Ayurvedic medicine for its ability to enhance energy, restore vitality, and promote overall health.

Unlike standard mineral supplements, Shilajit provides over 80 essential trace minerals, including magnesium, potassium, iron, zinc, and selenium, which are crucial for bone strength, fluid balance, energy production, and muscle function. What makes Shilajit truly exceptional is fulvic acid, a key compound that enhances mineral absorption at the cellular level, ensuring the body effectively utilizes these nutrients.

Beyond its mineral content, Shilajit is also a potent antioxidant, combating oxidative stress, reducing inflammation, and protecting mitochondria, the energy powerhouses of our cells. This dual-action of mineral replenishment and cellular defense makes Shilajit a foundational supplement for boosting energy, improving cognitive function, supporting heart health, and enhancing overall resilience. Whether you're looking to restore depleted nutrients, optimize energy levels, or strengthen the body's defense systems, Shilajit offers a science-backed solution that bridges ancient healing wisdom with modern health needs.

Science-Informed Shilajit Benefits

Supports Mitochondrial Energy and Reduces Fatigue

One of Shilajit's most studied functions is its ability to enhance mitochondrial function, the cellular structures responsible for producing energy (ATP). By improving the efficiency of energy production, Shilajit helps reduce physical fatigue and supports stamina and vitality. Fulvic acid, a primary active compound in Shilajit, also aids in transporting nutrients and oxygen into cells, further enhancing cellular energy metabolism. This makes Shilajit a supportive option for individuals experiencing low energy, general exhaustion, or conditions associated with mitochondrial decline.

Enhances Cognitive Function and Mental Clarity

Emerging research suggests that Shilajit may help protect brain cells against oxidative stress and support healthy neurological function. Fulvic acid has shown potential in breaking down abnormal tau proteins, structures implicated in neurodegenerative diseases such as Alzheimer's. Preliminary studies also suggest improvements in memory, focus, and mental clarity in individuals using Shilajit regularly. These effects are thought to be due to enhanced nutrient absorption, better cellular signaling, and reduced inflammation in neural tissue.

Promotes Healthy Aging and Cellular Protection

Oxidative stress is one of the primary biological processes that drive aging. Shilajit delivers a concentrated dose of natural antioxidants, which neutralize free radicals and help maintain cellular integrity. Additionally, it supports collagen production and may improve skin elasticity, helping to reduce visible signs of aging. Regular supplementation with Shilajit may assist in preserving resilience, vitality, and tissue repair as the body ages.

Supports Immune Function and Inflammatory Balance

Shilajit has been shown to help modulate immune responses by enhancing the activity of white blood cells and supporting the body's inflammatory pathways. Its high mineral content also plays a role in supporting immune defense. These effects contribute to better resistance to common illnesses and more efficient recovery from physical stress. Early studies suggest it may be useful in conditions marked by immune suppression or chronic low-grade inflammation.

Contributes to Hormonal Health and Male Fertility

Traditionally used to support male reproductive health, Shilajit has shown promising results in clinical studies focused on testosterone levels, sperm quality, and reproductive vitality. Research indicates improvements in sperm count, motility, and overall hormonal balance in men taking Shilajit consistently. These effects may be linked to its adaptogenic qualities and its support for endocrine system function.

Assists Liver Function and Natural Detoxification

Shilajit may support the body's natural detoxification processes by binding to heavy metals and environmental toxins, aiding their excretion through the liver and kidneys. Additionally, it has been observed to support liver cell regeneration and reduce oxidative damage in hepatic tissue. These effects may be especially relevant for individuals dealing with toxin exposure or liver health concerns related to inflammation or lifestyle factors.

Supports Joint Comfort and Mobility

Through its anti-inflammatory and antioxidant actions, Shilajit may help reduce joint stiffness and discomfort. It is thought to work by modulating inflammatory cytokines and supporting cartilage health. This makes it a potentially helpful addition to routines focused on joint comfort, especially in conditions such as osteoarthritis or age-related joint degeneration.

Enhances Physical Performance and Recovery

Athletes and physically active individuals may benefit from Shilajit's ability to increase mitochondrial efficiency and oxygen utilization. Some research suggests it may help reduce exercise-induced fatigue and support faster recovery by reducing inflammation and promoting tissue repair. These properties make Shilajit appealing for those looking to optimize endurance, strength, and post-exercise resilience.

Customer-Reported Shilajit Benefits

Shilajit has long been revered for its revitalizing potential, and modern users continue to echo that legacy through overwhelmingly positive real-world experiences. With an overall customer satisfaction rating of 4.3 out of 5, this mineral-rich adaptogen is especially valued for its ability to support natural energy levels, reduce inflammation, and restore mental clarity. Many users report noticeable improvements in stamina, joint comfort, and overall vitality, with several describing it as a life-changing addition to their wellness routine. Our analysis of verified customer reviews reveals key patterns in how Shilajit is being used and which benefits are most commonly reported.

Use Case Patterns Observed

Users turn to Shilajit for a diverse range of wellness goals, most commonly to increase energy, reduce inflammation, and support mental clarity. Many people with persistent fatigue, low stamina, or feelings of burnout found Shilajit appealing as a natural vitality booster. Those managing inflammation-related joint pain, especially in the knees or back, often reported trying it as an alternative to daily NSAIDs. Others shared that they began using Shilajit during high-stress periods or while managing hormonal fluctuations, hoping to restore a sense of balance and emotional steadiness. Some also incorporated Shilajit into broader wellness routines such as intermittent fasting, detoxification protocols, or post-viral fatigue recovery plans. A number of men also reported trying Shilajit to support testosterone levels or enhance reproductive health. Additionally, users struggling with brain fog, memory lapses, or mental sluggishness frequently cited improved cognitive focus as one of their primary goals for supplementing Shilajit.

Feedback Insights

Across thousands of positive reviews, users frequently described feeling a renewed sense of vitality, often within the first few days of use. Words like "energized," "clear-headed," and "rejuvenated" appear repeatedly, with several individuals noting a marked shift in both mood and stamina. One long-time user shared that after years of chronic fatigue and low motivation, Shilajit gave them "the fuel" to return to workouts and tackle long workdays with clarity and drive. Another reported that it helped lift the emotional fog that had lingered since a major illness, describing it as a turning point in both energy and outlook.

Users managing chronic inflammation or joint stiffness often described "night and day" differences in comfort and mobility. Several reported significant reductions in knee and back pain, even after years of relying on daily pain relievers. One user with post-surgical joint stiffness noted a dramatic return of flexibility and ease within just two days of use, while others described a newfound ability to move without discomfort. Although not everyone experienced fast results, many shared that with continued use, physical resilience, pain levels, and mood gradually improved.

Cognitive and emotional clarity were also recurring themes. Reviewers noted improvements in mental stamina, focus, and overall mood, often mentioning that they felt more grounded, calm, and motivated throughout the day. Some even reported improvements in sleep quality and a reduction in emotional swings, crediting Shilajit for helping to stabilize their nervous system.

Not all experiences were immediate or dramatic. A few reviewers mentioned that the benefits became more noticeable after a week or two of consistent use. Taste and smell were common points of complaint, but most agreed that the effects outweighed the inconvenience. Overall, users frequently expressed deep gratitude for discovering Shilajit, with several stating that it helped them reconnect with a version of themselves they hadn't felt in years.

Most Reported Benefits from Review Analysis

Shilajit is widely praised as a powerful revitalizing supplement, with many users calling it a game changer in their personal wellness routines. With an average rating of 4.3 out of 5 across tens of thousands of reviews, its reputation is backed not only by traditional use and modern science, but also by the lived experiences of real people. Our review analysis highlights which benefits customers report most often, giving you a practical window into how Shilajit may support your goals.

Each reported benefit reflects patterns seen repeatedly in user feedback. For example, 44 percent of reviewers described experiencing a noticeable boost in daily energy and vitality. Others frequently noted feeling calmer, sleeping more soundly, or experiencing improvements in sexual performance and cognitive clarity. These real-world insights help illustrate where Shilajit seems to have the strongest impact, based on what users most often say.

Below is a summary table of Shilajit's top benefits:

Benefit	%	Explanation
Energy Boost and Vitality	44%	Users frequently report feeling more energized, focused, and physically capable. Many describe this as a steady, sustained energy without a crash.
Stress, Anxiety, and Mood Support	25%	Shilajit is often associated with a calmer, more grounded mood. Users say they feel less overwhelmed and more emotionally resilient throughout the day.
Sleep Improvement	13%	Several reviewers note better quality sleep, fewer nighttime disruptions, and waking up feeling more rested and refreshed.
Sexual Health and Libido Support	10%	A number of men and women share that Shilajit enhances libido, performance, and overall intimacy, often in tandem with improved energy.
General Wellness and Mental Clarity	8%	Some users report better cognitive focus, reduced brain fog, and a general feeling of being more mentally sharp and physically balanced.

How to Use This Table

This table offers a practical guide based on the patterns observed in customer experience. If your main goal is to boost energy, it may be encouraging to see that this was the most frequently mentioned benefit, appearing in nearly half of all positive reviews. If you are seeking help with mood, stress, sleep, or focus, the data suggests many others have successfully used Shilajit for those outcomes as well.

Keep in mind that while every individual responds differently, the high percentage of satisfied users indicates that Shilajit holds strong potential across a variety of wellness goals. You can use this table to match your own priorities with the most commonly experienced benefits, helping you decide if this natural supplement aligns with your needs.

Application of Shilajit

Integrating Shilajit into your daily regimen is simple, especially with the convenience of capsules or tablets. These forms make it effortless to enjoy the benefits of Shilajit without the need for preparation. Capsules and tablets are pre-measured, portable, and easy to take, making them an excellent choice for busy lifestyles. Follow the manufacturer's dosage recommendations, typically ranging from 300 to 500 mg per day, and enjoy the convenience of adding this potent supplement to your routine with minimal effort.

For those who prefer variety, Shilajit also comes in resin and powdered forms. Pure Shilajit resin is the traditional option and can be dissolved in warm water, milk, or tea. While it offers an authentic experience, it requires more preparation. Powdered Shilajit, on the other hand, can be mixed into smoothies, juices, or other beverages for a customizable and easy-to-use alternative.

Probiotics

Your body is composed not only of trillions of human cells but also of a vast community of bacteria, viruses, fungi, and other microorganisms. These microbial cells may actually outnumber human cells, forming what scientists refer to as the human microbiome. Among the most well-known members of this community are probiotics, beneficial microbes that play important roles in digestion, immune regulation, and overall well-being.

Probiotics are friendly microorganisms, primarily specific strains of bacteria, that naturally live in harmony with your body. Most are found in the gut, which is often called the "second brain" due to its profound influence on mood, immune activity, and systemic inflammation. However, probiotics also reside in the mouth, skin, sinuses, and other mucosal areas, each with its own unique microbial environment.

When this internal ecosystem is balanced, with more beneficial microbes than harmful ones, many aspects of health tend to function more smoothly. Nutrient absorption improves, immune responses are well regulated, inflammation remains controlled, and the connection between the gut and brain functions more effectively. But when that balance is disrupted, whether by stress, medications, processed foods, or environmental toxins, the result can be a state known as dysbiosis. This imbalance may be associated with occasional digestive discomfort, recurring infections, skin issues, low energy, or changes in mood.

Probiotic supplements are designed to help maintain or restore microbial balance, especially after disruptions. Many contain well-studied strains such as *Lactobacillus*, *Bifidobacterium*, and *Saccharomyces boulardii*, which may support digestion, gut lining integrity, vitamin production, and microbial diversity.

Today, probiotics are increasingly appreciated not just for digestive support but also for their broader role in whole-body wellness. Their ability to support the immune system, encourage microbial harmony, and promote mental clarity makes them a valuable part of many long-term health routines.

In this chapter, you'll explore the science behind probiotic benefits, learn how different types of probiotics support the body, and discover what users commonly report from real-world experience.

Gut Probiotics and Mouth Probiotics

The Gut Microbiome: A Foundation of Health

The gut microbiome is an incredibly dynamic and complex system of microorganisms that influences digestion, immunity, mental focus, and metabolic balance. However, this system is easily disrupted by everyday factors like a high-sugar diet, antibiotics, lack of sleep, and chronic stress.

Gut probiotics are used to help restore balance in this environment by introducing beneficial microbes that may support healthy digestion, encourage a strong gut lining, and promote overall microbial diversity.

The Mouth Microbiome: A New Perspective on Oral Wellness

Traditional dental care often focuses on eliminating all bacteria. However, the mouth, like the gut, requires a balance of microbes to stay healthy. When beneficial oral bacteria are depleted, harmful ones may thrive, potentially contributing to gum issues, bad breath, or oral discomfort.

Instead of relying solely on harsh antiseptics, many people are turning to oral probiotics and natural dental care strategies to help support a balanced oral environment. A healthy oral microbiome may contribute not only to better gum and tooth health but also to reduced inflammation and a more holistic approach to dental care.

Creating a Supportive Environment for Probiotics

Even the highest quality probiotic strains may struggle to thrive if the gut environment is not supportive. A balanced digestive environment, rich in fiber, minerals, and hydration, helps good bacteria flourish. Without it, probiotics may have difficulty surviving or colonizing effectively.

For this reason, probiotic supplements are most effective when used as part of a broader wellness strategy. Supporting your gut with nourishing foods, stress management, and prebiotics creates the conditions these beneficial microbes need to do their best work.

Different Types of Probiotics

Not all probiotics function in the same way. The effectiveness of a probiotic supplement depends on its specific strains, their resilience, and their ability to survive stomach acid and reach their intended destination. Understanding the different categories of probiotics can help guide your selection based on your wellness goals.

Broad-Spectrum Gut Probiotics: *Lactobacillus* and *Bifidobacterium*

The most widely used and studied probiotics belong to the *Lactobacillus* and *Bifidobacterium* families. These strains are commonly used to support gut health, digestive function, and microbial balance. *Lactobacillus* species help break down food, produce lactic acid, and encourage a healthy environment within the gut. *Bifidobacterium* strains, which typically inhabit the large intestine, may help support regularity and promote a strong intestinal barrier. Blends containing both families are often used to support overall digestive wellness.

Spore-Based and Soil-Based Organisms (SBOs)

Spore-based and soil-based probiotics are naturally hardy strains found in the environment. These organisms, such as *Bacillus coagulans* and *Bacillus subtilis*, are known for their ability to survive extreme conditions, including stomach acid and heat. Because of this resilience, they are often selected by individuals looking for a more stable probiotic option. SBOs are commonly used to support digestive comfort, microbial diversity, and post-antibiotic recovery.

Targeted Strains for Specific Health Goals

Some probiotic strains are selected for more specific functions. For example, *Lactobacillus rhamnosus GG* has been studied for its potential role in supporting immune function and gastrointestinal balance during times of stress or travel. *Lactobacillus gasseri* has been explored for its possible influence on metabolism, and *Bifidobacterium breve* is often used in infant formulas to support early gut development. These targeted strains allow for more customized support, depending on individual health considerations.

Fermented Foods vs. Probiotic Supplements

Probiotics can come from both fermented foods and dietary supplements. Foods like yogurt, kefir, sauerkraut, kimchi, and kombucha naturally contain live microbes, along with enzymes and nutrients. These can be a great way to incorporate beneficial bacteria into your diet. However, probiotic content in foods may vary in strength and survivability. Supplements provide a consistent dose of specific strains that have often been clinically studied, which may be especially useful for individuals with digestive sensitivities or targeted wellness needs.

Oral Probiotics: Supporting Mouth and Throat Microbiomes

Oral probiotics are designed to support the balance of bacteria in the mouth, gums, and throat. Rather than acting on the gut, these strains are intended to help maintain a healthy oral environment. Strains like *Streptococcus salivarius* K12 and M18 have been studied for their ability to support oral hygiene, fresh breath, and microbial harmony in the upper respiratory tract. These are typically taken in lozenge or chewable form, which allows the strains to act locally in the mouth.

Understanding these categories can help you choose the probiotic approach that best aligns with your wellness goals, whether you're seeking digestive balance, immune support, or a more resilient oral environment.

Synergy with Foundational Natural Therapies

While probiotics offer important support on their own, they tend to work best when integrated into a broader wellness routine. Foundational natural therapies, such as herbal remedies, medicinal mushrooms, and nutrient-dense organ supplements, can create a more supportive environment for beneficial microbes to thrive.

Herbal Remedies

Herbs like ginger, licorice root, and peppermint are traditionally used to promote digestive comfort. These herbs may help soothe the gastrointestinal tract, reduce occasional bloating, and support healthy nutrient absorption, creating a gut environment where probiotics can flourish more effectively.

Medicinal Mushrooms

Mushrooms like Turkey Tail, Reishi, and Lion's Mane provide natural compounds that may help support immune function and microbial diversity. Many also contain prebiotic fibers, nutrients that feed beneficial bacteria. Incorporating these mushrooms into your routine can complement probiotic supplementation by enhancing gut ecology.

Beef Organ Supplements

Supplements made from nutrient-rich organs such as liver or spleen contain key vitamins and minerals that support digestive health. These include vitamin B12, iron, and amino acids that help maintain the integrity of the gut lining, which is crucial for creating a stable environment where probiotics can take hold.

By pairing probiotics with these supportive therapies, you help ensure that the internal terrain of your gut is well-prepared. When the environment is healthy, probiotics are more likely to colonize effectively, providing more consistent and lasting support for digestive wellness, immune resilience, and overall vitality.

Gut Probiotics

The human gut is more than just a site for digestion; it is a dynamic ecosystem that affects nearly every aspect of health. Within this environment lives a diverse population of microorganisms collectively known as the gut microbiome. This community includes trillions of bacteria, fungi, and other microbes that influence digestion, nutrient absorption, immune response, metabolic health, and even emotional well-being. Because of this wide-ranging impact, the gut is often referred to as the "second brain," highlighting its close connection to both the immune and nervous systems.

At the core of this system are probiotics, beneficial bacteria that help maintain microbial balance in the intestines. These microorganisms assist in breaking down food, producing vital nutrients like vitamin K and certain B vitamins, and supporting the integrity of the intestinal lining. They also play a defensive role by helping prevent overgrowth of harmful bacteria or yeast, especially after illness, stress, or antibiotic use.

However, maintaining a balanced gut microbiome has become increasingly challenging. Factors such as processed food, low-fiber diets, environmental toxins, chronic stress, and medications (particularly antibiotics) can disrupt the natural diversity of the gut. This disruption, known as dysbiosis, has been associated with a wide range of symptoms, including bloating, irregular bowel movements, food sensitivities, low energy, and frequent immune challenges.

Supplementing with gut probiotics offers a way to help restore and maintain a healthy internal environment. Commonly used strains such as *Lactobacillus* and *Bifidobacterium* have been extensively studied for their ability to support digestive comfort, immune function, and microbial balance. These supplements are particularly helpful for those experiencing digestive irregularities, recovering from antibiotic use, or simply looking to support long-term wellness through improved gut health.

In the sections that follow, we'll explore what scientific research reveals about the potential benefits of gut probiotics and examine what real-world users have consistently reported in their own health journeys. Together, these insights provide a well-rounded view of how gut probiotics may serve as a powerful tool in supporting your digestive and overall well-being.

Science-Informed Gut Probiotics Benefits

A growing body of research supports the role of gut probiotics in promoting digestive comfort, immune function, metabolic health, cognitive clarity, and the integrity of the gut lining. These beneficial bacteria help maintain a balanced gut ecosystem by supporting the natural diversity and function of the microbiome. Whether consumed through fermented foods or high-quality supplements, probiotics contribute to a healthier internal environment, which can enhance overall well-being and resilience.

Supports Digestive Comfort and Regularity

One of the most thoroughly studied benefits of probiotics is their impact on digestion. By assisting in the breakdown of food, probiotics can help reduce common symptoms such as bloating, gas, and occasional indigestion. They also promote smoother, more regular bowel movements, which may offer relief for those experiencing constipation or irregularity. Specific strains, including species from the *Lactobacillus* and *Bifidobacterium* families, have demonstrated the ability to support intestinal motility and improve stool consistency. In individuals with occasional digestive discomfort, these strains may help ease abdominal pressure and encourage a more balanced digestive rhythm. A meta-analysis published in *The American Journal of Clinical Nutrition* reported consistent improvement in stool regularity and digestive symptoms among participants using targeted probiotic formulas.

Supports a Balanced Immune Response

Approximately 70 percent of the body's immune cells are located in the gut. This close connection allows probiotics to influence immune regulation by helping maintain the microbiome's balance and by interacting with gut-associated lymphoid tissue (GALT). Several probiotic strains have been shown to support immune resilience by enhancing the body's natural antibody production and promoting a well-coordinated immune response. They may also help restore microbial balance following antibiotic use, which can be particularly important for minimizing occasional digestive upset and reducing the risk of microbial imbalance. In a study published in *The Journal of Science and Medicine in Sport*, athletes who took probiotics experienced fewer upper respiratory symptoms and demonstrated stronger immune markers during training.

Contributes to Metabolic Health and Nutrient Processing

Emerging research suggests that probiotics may play a supportive role in metabolic function. Certain strains have been studied for their potential to promote healthy weight maintenance and body composition. For instance, *Lactobacillus gasseri* has been associated with modest reductions in waist circumference and visceral fat when taken consistently. Additionally, the gut microbiome plays a role in processing carbohydrates and regulating insulin sensitivity. By supporting microbial balance, probiotics may help maintain more stable blood sugar responses and lipid metabolism. Clinical reviews in *Obesity Reviews* and other journals suggest that regular probiotic intake may contribute to metabolic balance, especially when combined with a nutrient-rich diet and active lifestyle.

Supports the Gut-Brain Connection and Emotional Well-Being

The relationship between the gut and the brain, often referred to as the gut-brain axis, is increasingly recognized as a key factor in emotional and cognitive health. The microbiome influences the production of neurotransmitters, such as serotonin and gamma-aminobutyric acid (GABA), which play roles in mood regulation and emotional stability. Probiotic supplementation has been associated with improved emotional resilience, reduced feelings of stress, and better cognitive performance. In a study published in *Frontiers in Psychiatry*, individuals who took a multi-strain probiotic reported improvements in emotional balance and mental clarity compared to a placebo group. While individual responses vary, these findings suggest that a healthy gut microbiome may contribute to a more centered and focused state of mind.

Helps Maintain Gut Barrier Function

The integrity of the gut lining is essential for nutrient absorption and for preventing the movement of unwanted substances into the bloodstream. When the barrier becomes compromised, it can contribute to increased intestinal permeability, sometimes referred to as "leaky gut." Probiotics help support this protective function by encouraging the growth of beneficial bacteria, stimulating the production of mucosal lining, and enhancing the function of tight junction proteins between intestinal cells. Specific strains, such as *Lactobacillus rhamnosus* and *Bifidobacterium lactis*, have been studied for their ability to promote gut barrier stability. A review in the journal

Nutrients found that probiotic supplementation may contribute to improved gut integrity and reduced inflammatory signaling in individuals with digestive sensitivities.

Customer-Reported Gut Probiotics Benefits

Probiotics have become one of the most trusted wellness tools for people dealing with digestive discomfort, bloating, immune challenges, and gut-related fatigue. While clinical research continues to validate their many benefits, it is the personal experiences of real users that bring these benefits to life. With an impressive overall customer satisfaction rating of 4.5 out of 5 stars, gut probiotics are consistently praised for their ability to help people feel lighter, more regular, and more balanced, physically, emotionally, and even mentally.

These reviews reflect a common theme: when gut health improves, so does quality of life. Whether recovering from antibiotic use, trying to manage IBS symptoms, or simply hoping to improve daily digestion, users often describe probiotics as a turning point in their wellness journey. For many, they are no longer just a supplement but a daily essential.

Use Case Patterns Observed

The most common reason people begin taking gut probiotics is to find relief from persistent digestive issues such as bloating, constipation, gas, and irregular bowel movements. Many users mention long-standing struggles with IBS, GERD, or sluggish digestion and report that probiotic supplementation helped them regain regularity and comfort in a way other remedies could not.

Another major pattern involves recovery and rebuilding after antibiotic use or gastrointestinal distress, including traveler's diarrhea. These users were seeking to restore microbial balance, reduce symptoms of discomfort, and support the healing process. Several also note that probiotics helped manage sugar cravings and supported their metabolism during weight management or dietary changes.

For women, hormonal balance and vaginal health are often key drivers. Many selected formulas designed specifically for women and noted improvements not only in digestion but also in PMS symptoms, odor control, and yeast balance.

In more targeted cases, some users reported using probiotics to support cholesterol management, improve skin conditions like rosacea and acne, reduce arthritis-related inflammation, and even maintain cognitive clarity during early memory decline.

Across all cases, people who added probiotics to their wellness routines often did so after trying many other interventions, sometimes even prescription medications, with little success. Their motivation is often driven by a desire for a natural, effective solution that promotes internal balance.

Feedback Insights

What stands out most in the feedback is the strong emotional relief people express after finally finding something that works. Many use phrases like "game-changer," "life-changing," or "the only thing that helped me" when describing the impact probiotics had on their daily well-being.

A large number of users shared that they felt "lighter," "less bloated," and "more regular" within the first week. One reviewer noted that they had tried everything for IBS-related discomfort, but only probiotics delivered reliable results. Another shared that their lifelong constipation and painful bloating disappeared after just a few days on a new probiotic regimen, something they hadn't achieved even with specialized medications.

Many emphasized how probiotics gave them back a sense of control. One person described feeling "confident enough to eat again while traveling" after overcoming recurring bouts of traveler's diarrhea. Another shared that they no longer feared meals or unexpected flare-ups at work thanks to newfound digestive stability.

Even emotional well-being surfaced as a recurring theme. Several users reported feeling less anxious, less foggy, and more emotionally stable after restoring their gut balance. One reviewer specifically credited probiotics with helping regulate their mood during hormonal shifts and another expressed surprise at how quickly their cravings diminished and energy levels improved.

The sense of gratitude is strong across the board. For some, probiotics helped them avoid prescription medications. For others, they became a foundation for healing after years of physical discomfort. Even when reviewers admitted initial skepticism, their final verdict was often a firm commitment to keep probiotics as part of their daily health routine.

Most Reported Benefits from Review Analysis

Gut probiotics continue to earn strong support from real users seeking relief from digestive discomfort, immune challenges, and low energy. With an overall rating of 4.5 out of 5 stars, these supplements are consistently praised for helping people feel lighter, more regular, and better balanced, both physically and emotionally. Customer feedback highlights just how impactful probiotic therapy can be, especially for those struggling with bloating, constipation, or an unpredictable digestive system.

After analyzing thousands of verified reviews, five major benefit categories emerged. These benefits reflect the real-world experiences of users who found measurable improvements in their gut health and quality of life after starting probiotic supplements. While individual results may vary, the percentages below give a clear picture of which outcomes were most commonly reported.

Below is a summary table of the most frequently mentioned benefits, based on positive customer experiences:

Below is a summary of Gut Probiotics' top benefits as reported by customers:

Benefit	%	Explanation
Digestion Support	42%	Users frequently describe easier digestion, reduced discomfort after meals, and better nutrient absorption. Many mention relief from heartburn, gas, and indigestion.
Regularity Improvement	21%	Helps promote more consistent bowel movements, reducing issues like constipation, urgency, or unpredictable cycles.
Bloating Relief	16%	Many users report feeling lighter and less bloated, especially after eating. Probiotics appear to help reduce excess gas and digestive swelling.
Immune System Boost	11%	Several reviewers noted fewer colds and quicker recovery, especially after antibiotics or seasonal illnesses.
Energy and Well-Being	8%	Some users noticed a boost in energy, mental clarity, and overall resilience after rebalancing their gut microbiome.

How to Use This Table

Start by identifying the health goals that matter most to you. If digestion is a top concern, for example, take note that digestion support was the most commonly reported benefit, mentioned in 42% of positive reviews. This means that people with similar concerns often found meaningful improvement after adding gut probiotics to their routine.

Each percentage represents the proportion of users who voluntarily mentioned that specific benefit in a positive review. Higher numbers suggest stronger patterns across a broad base of experiences. However, it's important to remember that everyone's body is different. What works well for one person may take more time or require a different strain for another.

These findings are not clinical outcomes, but they do offer valuable insights from real people who were looking for the same kinds of relief. Whether you're seeking more regularity, fewer digestive disruptions, or better overall well-being, gut probiotics are a widely trusted and well-reviewed choice that many users rely on daily.

Application of Gut Probiotics

Adding gut probiotics to your daily routine can be a simple and rewarding step toward better digestive health and overall well-being. Probiotic supplements are widely available in convenient formats such as capsules, chewables, powders, and liquid drops. This flexibility makes it easy to choose a form that fits your preferences and lifestyle, whether you prefer to take your supplements with meals, on the go, or as part of your morning or evening wellness routine.

If you're new to probiotics, it's best to begin with a lower dose and give your body time to adjust. As probiotics begin to repopulate your gut with beneficial bacteria, you may notice subtle changes in digestion or bowel habits. These early shifts are typically temporary and may be part of your microbiome adapting to the new balance. After a few days or weeks, many people find that their digestive system feels more comfortable, regular, and resilient.

Consistency is key. Unlike some supplements that can be taken occasionally, probiotics work best when used daily. The gut microbiome is a living system that benefits from regular nourishment. Skipping doses or using them inconsistently may reduce their effectiveness. For the best results, follow the instructions provided on the product label, or speak with a qualified healthcare practitioner to determine the right strain and dosage for your specific health needs.

To enhance the effectiveness of probiotic supplements, consider pairing them with prebiotics, the fibers and plant compounds that feed and support beneficial gut bacteria. Prebiotics can be found in a variety of fiber-rich foods, including garlic, onions, leeks, bananas, oats, and asparagus. You can also supplement prebiotics through options like psyllium husk or inulin, which create an ideal environment for probiotics to flourish.

For individuals managing digestive concerns, combining probiotics with a balanced diet, adequate hydration, and a steady sleep routine can further support a healthy microbiome. Over time, this integrated approach can help maintain regularity, reduce bloating, and promote more stable energy levels.

Ultimately, probiotics are not a quick fix but a valuable part of a longer-term strategy for digestive wellness. With consistent use and the right support, they can play a central role in creating a stronger, healthier gut, and by extension, a healthier you.

Oral Probiotics

When most people think of probiotics, they think of gut health. But the mouth has its own thriving microbiome, one that plays a critical role in oral hygiene, immune defense, and even whole-body health. This complex microbial community helps regulate the balance between beneficial and harmful bacteria in the mouth, directly influencing the health of the teeth, gums, sinuses, throat, and beyond.

Oral probiotics are designed to support this delicate ecosystem. Unlike gut probiotics, which target the digestive tract, oral probiotics introduce specific strains of beneficial bacteria that colonize the mouth and upper respiratory tract. These strains help inhibit the growth of odor-causing and pathogenic bacteria, support gum and throat health, and contribute to fresher breath and a stronger immune barrier at one of the body's primary points of entry.

Emerging research also suggests connections between the oral microbiome and broader aspects of health, including cognitive function, heart health, and the gut-brain axis. By nurturing a healthy microbial balance in the mouth, oral probiotics offer a proactive and natural way to protect not only dental wellness but also systemic health.

In the sections ahead, we'll explore what the science says about oral probiotics and how real-world users are benefiting from this increasingly popular approach to foundational self-care.

Science-Informed Oral Probiotics Benefits

Scientific understanding of the oral microbiome continues to grow, revealing its critical role in supporting not only dental health but also broader aspects of immunity and systemic wellness. Oral probiotics offer a proactive and natural way to support this complex ecosystem by promoting beneficial bacteria and reducing the overgrowth of problematic strains. These effects can help improve gum health, freshen breath, reduce the risk of cavities, and support throat and respiratory health, without disrupting the natural balance of the mouth.

Supports Gum Health and Helps Maintain Periodontal Wellness

The gums are especially sensitive to microbial imbalance. When harmful bacteria accumulate along the gumline, they can trigger inflammation, tissue damage, and eventually lead to periodontal issues such as gingivitis or periodontitis. Certain probiotic strains, including *Lactobacillus reuteri* and *Streptococcus salivarius K12*, have demonstrated the ability to promote healthy microbial communities in the mouth while reducing markers associated with gum inflammation.

Clinical research has shown that individuals supplementing these strains may experience reductions in gum bleeding, plaque accumulation, and the presence of bacteria associated with gum disease. A study published in *The Journal of Clinical Periodontology* found that individuals taking *Lactobacillus reuteri* saw measurable improvements in gum health, including reduced inflammation and more stable oral microbial profiles.

Helps Reduce Bad Breath by Balancing Oral Bacteria

Chronic bad breath, or halitosis, is frequently caused by volatile sulfur compounds (VSCs) produced by odor-causing bacteria. While mouthwashes and breath-freshening products may offer short-term masking, they often fail to address the underlying microbial imbalance. Oral probiotics provide a more sustainable approach by encouraging a healthier balance of microorganisms in the mouth.

One of the most well-studied strains for this purpose is *Streptococcus salivarius K12*, which has been shown to reduce the populations of VSC-producing bacteria. In a study published in *Applied and Environmental Microbiology*, participants taking *S. salivarius K12* reported significantly improved breath freshness along with measurable reductions in oral VSC levels. These findings support the use of probiotics as a long-term tool for managing oral odor by restoring balance at the microbial level.

Supports Tooth Health and Helps Reduce the Risk of Cavities

Dental cavities form when acids produced by certain bacteria, such as *Streptococcus mutans*, erode the protective enamel on teeth. Oral probiotics can help reduce the activity of these bacteria by introducing strains that compete with or inhibit their growth. Strains such as *Lactobacillus paracasei* and *Lactobacillus rhamnosus* have demonstrated potential to lower acid production, reduce plaque formation, and support overall oral cleanliness.

In research published in *Caries Research*, individuals who supplemented with probiotic strains targeting oral health showed decreased levels of *S. mutans* in their saliva. This reduction suggests a decreased risk of enamel erosion and tooth decay over time, particularly when paired with regular brushing and dental care.

Supports Throat Immunity and Upper Respiratory Defense

The benefits of oral probiotics are not limited to the teeth and gums. The upper respiratory tract shares microbial communities with the mouth, and probiotic strains that colonize this area can help strengthen immune responses to common infections. Strains like

Streptococcus salivarius K12 and *S. salivarius M18* have been studied for their ability to support throat and sinus health.

These probiotics work by producing natural antibacterial substances that help reduce the presence of harmful pathogens in the throat, thereby supporting the body's natural defenses. A study in *Pediatrics* found that children who took *S. salivarius K12* experienced fewer episodes of sore throat and ear infections, indicating a potential role for probiotics in immune support beyond the digestive system.

Promotes Long-Term Oral Microbiome Balance

A healthy oral microbiome relies on the presence of diverse and well-regulated microbial populations. Disruption to this balance, whether from antibiotics, poor diet, or overuse of antiseptic products, can lead to recurring dental and gum issues. Oral probiotics help restore harmony by promoting beneficial bacteria that contribute to oral tissue integrity, reduce inflammation, and protect against overgrowth of problematic species.

Importantly, oral probiotics do not sterilize the mouth. Instead, they encourage a natural balance that supports both local and systemic health. Research in *The Journal of Oral Microbiology* has highlighted that a stable oral microbiome is associated with a lower risk of developing systemic conditions that have been linked to poor oral health, including cardiovascular concerns and metabolic imbalances.

Oral Probiotics and Brain Health

The oral microbiome plays a far-reaching role in health, extending its influence well beyond the mouth. Emerging research suggests that imbalances in oral bacteria may contribute to systemic inflammation and have implications for cognitive health. Scientists have observed associations between oral bacterial activity and conditions such as cognitive decline, dementia, and Alzheimer's disease. Oral probiotics support microbial balance in the mouth, which may help reduce these risks and promote long-term neurological well-being.

Helps Reduce Inflammation That May Affect Cognitive Function

Persistent inflammation in the body is widely recognized as a contributing factor to cognitive aging and neurodegeneration. Poor oral health, including conditions like gingivitis and periodontitis, can introduce low-grade, chronic inflammation that spreads beyond the oral cavity. This systemic inflammation has been linked in several studies to accelerated cognitive decline. Oral probiotics may assist in maintaining a balanced microbial community, which in turn may help reduce inflammatory markers and support a more favorable internal environment for brain health.

May Help Limit the Spread of Harmful Bacteria

Research has identified certain oral bacteria, such as *Porphyromonas gingivalis*, in the brain tissue of individuals with neurodegenerative conditions. These bacteria are known to contribute to gum disease and may enter the bloodstream or access neural pathways. Although more research is needed to fully understand this connection, maintaining a healthy oral microbiome may help reduce the spread of these microbes. Oral probiotics may support this balance by discouraging the overgrowth of inflammatory strains and helping sustain the protective microbial populations within the mouth.

Supports Nitric Oxide Production and Brain Circulation

The oral microbiome is also involved in converting dietary nitrates into nitric oxide, a compound that supports blood flow, including to the brain. Nitric oxide helps regulate vascular tone, enhance oxygen delivery, and reduce oxidative stress in the nervous system. Disruptions in oral microbial balance may impair this conversion process. Certain probiotic strains may help maintain a healthier environment for nitrate reduction, supporting nitric oxide levels and contributing to brain oxygenation and circulation.

May Contribute to Reduced Stroke and Cardiovascular Risk

Several studies have linked poor oral health to increased risk of cardiovascular events, including stroke, an event that can impact memory, cognition, and overall brain performance. Some oral bacteria have been associated with inflammation in blood vessels and the development of arterial plaque. By helping to maintain a balanced oral microbiome, probiotics may support healthier blood vessel function and reduce factors that contribute to cardiovascular strain. These effects may, over time, play a role in protecting the brain from vascular-related damage.

Customer-Reported Oral Probiotics Benefits

Oral probiotics have gained a loyal following among individuals seeking fresher breath, healthier gums, and a more balanced oral environment. With an overall satisfaction rating of 4.2 out of 5 stars, these supplements are often described as a small daily habit that makes a noticeable difference in both comfort and confidence. While many people are familiar with probiotics for digestive health, oral probiotics are specifically formulated to support the unique bacterial ecosystem of the mouth, gums, throat, and sinuses. Our analysis of verified customer reviews reveals how these supplements are being used in real life, why people turn to them, what they hope to resolve, and how they describe the results. The insights that follow are drawn from individuals who rated their experiences positively and often shared compelling, heartfelt accounts of how oral probiotics helped them regain control of their oral health and overall well-being.

Use Case Patterns Observed

Oral probiotics are most commonly used by people who have long struggled with bad breath, bleeding gums, gum recession, or recurring sore throats. Many users had already tried conventional strategies, specialty toothpaste, antiseptic rinses, rigorous brushing and flossing, yet still felt dissatisfied. A large number turned to oral probiotics after learning more about the importance of maintaining a balanced oral microbiome. For some, this shift came after repeated courses of antibiotics, radiation treatment, or hormonal changes that disrupted their oral health. Parents often purchased these probiotics for children with chronic strep infections or throat discomfort, while adults frequently sought support for gum sensitivity, plaque control, or dry mouth during Invisalign or post-dental work. In several cases, users chose oral probiotics as a daily preventive measure to complement their oral hygiene routines and protect against deeper systemic health concerns.

Feedback Insights

Customer feedback often reflects a sense of both relief and surprise. Many people weren't sure what to expect, and were genuinely impressed by the results. One user shared that even after extensive dental hygiene, they still struggled with chronic bad breath until oral probiotics "completely changed everything." Others described regaining confidence in social situations after years of discomfort, noting that their breath felt fresh even in the mornings or after long periods without brushing.

Several users described physical improvements that went beyond breath, including less gum bleeding, reduced pocket depth scores during dental exams, and even signs of gum tissue regrowth. Others mentioned waking up with noticeably cleaner mouths and less plaque buildup, with some saying they had postponed or avoided invasive dental treatments thanks to consistent probiotic use. Oral cancer survivors and those recovering from long-term antibiotic use often emphasized how helpful these supplements were in soothing inflammation, promoting healing, and making oral care feel more manageable again.

There was also a significant emotional dimension in many reviews. Parents expressed deep gratitude after seeing their children experience fewer sore throats or less teasing at school due to halitosis. Adults who had felt embarrassed or defeated by ongoing oral discomfort described these probiotics as "life-changing," "a miracle," or simply "worth every penny." Across all groups, the tone was overwhelmingly positive, with users frequently reporting that oral probiotics had become a trusted and permanent part of their daily health rituals.

Most Reported Benefits from Review Analysis

Oral probiotics have received wide appreciation from customers seeking natural ways to support breath freshness, gum health, and oral microbiome balance. With an overall customer satisfaction rating of 4.2 out of 5 stars, many users report noticeable improvements in how their mouth feels, looks, and functions. These benefits are especially valued by individuals who had tried conventional oral care routines, brushing, flossing, mouthwash, yet still struggled with persistent issues like gum sensitivity, bad breath, or recurring plaque buildup.

Our analysis of verified, positively rated reviews reveals clear patterns in what users found most helpful. Each percentage shown below reflects how often that benefit was mentioned among those who had a successful experience with oral probiotic supplements. A higher percentage suggests that people with similar concerns may be more likely to experience similar results.

For example, if 33% of reviewers mentioned overall oral health improvements, it suggests that one in three people felt meaningful change in their dental hygiene routine, gum comfort, or tooth cleanliness after using these supplements.

Below is a summary of Oral Probiotics' top benefits as reported by customers:

Benefit	%	Explanation
Overall oral health	33%	Many users reported better checkups, cleaner teeth, less plaque, and fresh breath.
Bad breath reduction	27%	Users noticed a major improvement in breath freshness, often described as "life-changing."
Gum health improvement	20%	Reports include healthier gums, less bleeding, less swelling, and reduced sensitivity.
Cavity and plaque support	12%	Several users observed reduced tartar buildup and less concern about new cavities.
Throat and sinus support	7%	Some individuals experienced fewer sore throats and improved sinus comfort.

How to Use This Table

This summary provides a quick snapshot of the most common user-reported benefits of oral probiotics. It is not intended as a guarantee, but rather as a reflection of what real people have experienced after consistent use. If your goals align with the top-reported categories, such as improving gum comfort or reducing bad breath, these insights may help you decide whether oral probiotics are a good fit for your personal oral care routine. Keep in mind that results vary depending on your existing health, habits, and how consistently the supplement is used.

With continued research and real-world feedback, oral probiotics are gaining attention as a meaningful, natural addition to modern oral hygiene. For many people, they have become a valued daily habit that helps restore confidence and comfort from the inside out.

Application of Oral Probiotics

Oral probiotics are typically available in the form of chewable tablets or lozenges designed to dissolve slowly in the mouth. Unlike digestive probiotics, which target the gut, oral probiotics work best when given direct contact with the tissues of the mouth, gums, and throat. To maximize their effectiveness, allow the tablet to fully dissolve without chewing or swallowing it whole. This ensures that the beneficial bacteria have time to colonize the oral cavity and support a healthier microbiome.

For best results, take oral probiotics after brushing and flossing, ideally at night before bed or in the morning after your first oral hygiene routine. Avoid eating or drinking for at least 30 minutes after taking the probiotic to allow the beneficial strains time to settle in. Consistency is key. Regular use supports a stable microbial environment that can reduce unwanted bacteria and promote lasting oral health.

Always follow the instructions provided on the product label or consult your healthcare provider for guidance, especially if you have underlying dental conditions or sensitivities.

Although not required, some people find additional benefit by supporting their oral microbiome with a clean, low-sugar diet and the use of oral prebiotics when available. These may help feed and sustain the beneficial bacteria introduced by the probiotic, encouraging a more resilient oral environment.

With proper use, oral probiotics can become a simple but powerful addition to your daily wellness routine, helping you maintain fresher breath, healthier gums, and a more balanced oral ecosystem.

Enzymes

Enzymes are the invisible drivers behind nearly every function in your body. They are biological catalysts, specialized proteins that spark and accelerate the chemical reactions needed for life. Without enzymes, essential processes such as digestion, energy production, cellular repair, and immune defense simply wouldn't occur. Every moment, millions of enzymatic reactions are happening throughout your body, working silently to keep you alive and well.

Enzymes play a crucial role in breaking down the food you eat into absorbable nutrients. They convert carbohydrates into sugars, proteins into amino acids, and fats into fatty acids so your body can absorb and utilize them for energy, repair, and growth. Beyond digestion, enzymes regulate metabolism, assist in detoxifying harmful substances, repair damaged DNA, reduce inflammation, and support immune function. They are vital not only for digestion but also for maintaining cellular health and longevity.

There are three primary types of enzymes that impact human health: digestive enzymes that help break down food in your stomach and intestines, metabolic enzymes that work within your cells to carry out energy production and detoxification, and food-based enzymes naturally present in raw fruits, vegetables, and fermented foods. Unfortunately, modern diets high in processed, cooked, and enzyme-depleted foods place significant stress on your digestive system. Over time, this can lead to sluggish digestion, poor nutrient absorption, bloating, fatigue, and systemic inflammation. This is where enzyme supplementation becomes essential.

Digestive enzyme supplements provide targeted support by helping your body break down macronutrients in meals. Whether you're eating protein, fats, starches, or fiber-rich vegetables, these enzymes help ensure your digestive process is smooth, efficient, and comfortable. They can also help reduce symptoms like indigestion, gas, bloating, and discomfort after meals. For individuals with low stomach acid, gallbladder dysfunction, or pancreatic enzyme insufficiency, digestive enzyme support may be especially beneficial. In these cases, supplementation not only relieves symptoms but also supports better nutrient absorption, which is foundational for health.

Each enzyme plays a specific role in the breakdown of macronutrients. Proteases help break down proteins into amino acids, which are essential for muscle growth, immune defense, hormone production, and tissue repair. Lipases assist in digesting fats into fatty acids and glycerol, supporting energy metabolism and the absorption of fat-soluble vitamins. Amylases help convert carbohydrates into simple sugars for energy, and cellulases work to digest plant fibers, making it easier to extract nutrients from high-fiber foods. When any of these enzymes are lacking, digestive strain and nutrient imbalances can occur. Supplementing with the right combination can offer both immediate and long-term benefits.

There are four main categories of digestive enzyme support, each with distinct benefits. The first is Pancreatin, a concentrated enzyme blend extracted from the pancreas of animals that mimics the body's natural enzyme output. Pancreatin is particularly useful for individuals who struggle with digesting proteins and fats, and it can significantly reduce bloating and discomfort after meals.

The second option includes plant-based and fungal-derived enzymes. These are ideal for individuals following plant-based diets or those who prefer non-animal sources. Common examples include bromelain from pineapple, papain from papaya, and fungal-based proteases and cellulases. These enzymes are gentle, broad-spectrum, and well tolerated by most individuals.

The third solution is Betaine Hydrochloride (HCL), which supports healthy stomach acid levels. Although not an enzyme itself, Betaine HCL plays a critical role in activating pepsin, an enzyme necessary for protein digestion. Many people suffer from low stomach acid without realizing it, and restoring proper acidity is often the missing key to solving chronic digestive issues.

Finally, beef organ supplements offer a dual benefit: they provide natural enzymes directly from nutrient-dense organs like the pancreas and stomach while simultaneously nourishing the body's own enzyme-producing systems. This approach not only offers digestive support but also helps restore the body's natural digestive capacity over time.

Beef organ supplements are briefly introduced here, as extensive information is available in the book *Animal Organ Therapy*, part of *The Medicine-Free, Illness-Free Series*. The chapters that follow will explore Betaine HCL, Pancreatin, and Plant-Based Enzymes in greater detail.

By choosing the approach that best suits your needs, whether enzyme replacement, digestive stimulation, or organ support, you can restore digestive ease and improve nutrient utilization across the board. In the sections that follow, we will explore each of these digestive enzyme strategies in greater depth to help you decide which solution, or combination of solutions, is best for your unique health goals.

Enzyme-Rich Beef Organ Supplements

Beef organ supplements, derived from nutrient-dense organs such as the pancreas, gallbladder, spleen, and stomach, offer a unique and natural source of digestive enzymes. Unlike conventional enzyme supplements that act as a direct replacement, beef organ supplements provide dual benefits: they supply digestive enzymes while also nourishing the body's enzyme-producing organs. This means they support your body in regaining its own enzyme production capabilities rather than creating dependency.

These supplements deliver animal-based enzymes tailored to digestive needs. The pancreas contributes proteases and lipases for protein and fat digestion, while the gallbladder supplies bile acids to emulsify fats. The spleen supports immune function and the breakdown of old red blood cells, and the stomach provides pepsinogen, essential for efficient protein digestion. By targeting specific macronutrients, these enzymes can alleviate common digestive issues like bloating, gas, and indigestion.

What sets beef organ supplements apart is their ability to nourish corresponding human organs, promoting long-term digestive health. For example, consuming pancreas supplement supports the health and function of your pancreas, enhancing its natural enzyme production. This dual-action approach ensures sustained digestive efficiency and reinforces gut health, rather than merely substituting what the body should produce.

Additionally, these supplements improve nutrient absorption, ensuring the body receives essential vitamins and minerals for overall vitality. They also play a key role in energy production and metabolic regulation, helping to maintain steady energy levels. Beyond digestion, the enzymes in beef organ supplements support immune function by aiding detoxification and nutrient availability, strengthening the body's resilience against infections.

Beef organ supplements are a compelling choice for those seeking a natural, comprehensive approach to digestive and systemic health. Rich in bioavailable nutrients and digestive-supporting compounds, certain beef organs contain natural enzymes, bile acids, and cofactors that aid in nutrient absorption and gut function.

Beef pancreas is a primary source of digestive enzymes, including lipase, protease, and amylase, which support the breakdown of fats, proteins, and carbohydrates.

Beef liver provides essential cofactors like vitamin B12 and choline, which enhance metabolic and digestive processes.

Beef stomach (tripe) contains intrinsic factor, crucial for vitamin B12 absorption, while beef intestines supply key peptides and probiotics that support gut flora balance.

Ox bile and gallbladder are rich in bile acids, which aid in fat digestion, absorption of fat-soluble vitamins (A, D, E, K), and liver detoxification. These play a vital role in maintaining healthy digestion and preventing fat malabsorption issues.

By supporting rather than replacing the body's own functions, beef organ supplements provide lasting benefits for gut health, energy, and immunity, making them a foundational addition to a digestive wellness regimen.

For more information about Beef Organ Supplement for Digestive Enzymes, please refer to the *Animal Organ Therapy*.

Betaine Hydrochloride (Betaine HCL)

While digestive enzymes and beef organ supplements help break down food, they require the right environment to work effectively. That environment is created by stomach acid, and for many people, especially those with chronic digestive discomfort, acid levels may be too low. Betaine Hydrochloride (Betaine HCL) is a naturally derived compound that helps restore healthy stomach acidity, setting the stage for more complete digestion and better nutrient absorption.

Low stomach acid is more common than most people think. It can contribute to bloating, heaviness after meals, poor protein breakdown, and even nutrient deficiencies. These issues are particularly common in individuals over 40 or those following high-protein diets such as Paleo or Carnivore. In such cases, supplementing Betaine HCL can ease discomfort and help the digestive process function more efficiently.

One of the most misunderstood conditions linked to low stomach acid is acid reflux. Although it seems logical to blame reflux on too much acid, research and clinical experience suggest the opposite may be true: reflux can occur when there is not enough acid to maintain proper closure of the lower esophageal sphincter. Supporting acidity with Betaine HCL may help reduce reflux by restoring normal digestive signaling and tone.

Importantly, Betaine HCL is not intended as a permanent replacement for your body's own acid production. It is best used as a temporary tool to support digestion while encouraging the stomach to “wake up” and resume its natural function. Many people find that after a few weeks or months, they can taper off the supplement as their digestion improves. This makes Betaine HCL not only effective but also empowering as part of a long-term healing approach.

In the sections that follow, we'll explore the science behind how Betaine HCL supports digestive health and review real-world feedback from individuals who have found relief using this simple, targeted supplement.

Science-Informed Betaine HCL Benefits

Enhances Protein Digestion and Nutrient Absorption

Betaine HCL supports the digestive process by increasing stomach acidity, which is essential for the activation of pepsin, the enzyme that breaks proteins into absorbable amino acids. When stomach acid is insufficient, protein digestion becomes impaired, which can lead to feelings of fullness, gas, or discomfort after meals. In this low-acid state, the body may also struggle to absorb key nutrients such as calcium, magnesium, iron, zinc, and vitamins B12 and C, all of which require an acidic environment for optimal absorption. Supplementing Betaine HCL helps restore the acidic conditions needed for digestive efficiency, making it especially useful for those who feel they are not getting the most from their food despite eating well.

Supports a Balanced Gut Environment and Microbial Health

Stomach acid is not only important for digestion, it also serves as a natural defense system. A well-acidified stomach helps limit the survival of harmful microorganisms that can disrupt the balance of gut flora. When acid levels are low, undigested food tends to remain in the stomach longer than it should, encouraging fermentation and increasing the risk of gas, bloating, and bacterial overgrowth in the small intestine. Research has shown that increasing stomach acidity with Betaine HCL can help reduce the risk of microbial imbalance and support a healthier digestive environment. This makes it a valuable tool for those concerned about occasional digestive upset or microbial overgrowth linked to low acid levels.

Supports Comfortable Digestion and Helps Reduce Reflux Associated with Low Acid

While reflux is often attributed to excess acid, low stomach acid can also be a contributing factor. When acid production is insufficient, the lower esophageal sphincter (LES), which acts as a valve between the stomach and esophagus, may lose proper tone, allowing partially digested food and stomach contents to move upward. Betaine HCL may help restore the acidic conditions that support LES function, making it less likely for reflux to occur. For individuals who experience occasional acid reflux symptoms despite eating clean or avoiding common triggers, low acid could be a hidden factor. Supporting normal acidity levels with Betaine HCL can promote more comfortable digestion and reduce the chance of unwanted backflow into the esophagus.

Supports Meat Digestion and High-Protein Diets

For individuals who follow protein-rich eating styles such as Paleo, Carnivore, or Keto diets, adequate stomach acid is especially important. Proteins and fats take more digestive effort to break down than simple carbohydrates, and they require a highly acidic environment to initiate that process. Without it, meals heavy in meat may lead to a feeling of heaviness, sluggishness, or digestive discomfort. Betaine HCL supports the digestive breakdown of protein and fat, improving meal tolerance and helping the body better access the nutrients found in meat and other dense foods. For those who enjoy meat-centric meals but experience discomfort afterward, Betaine HCL can offer meaningful digestive support.

Customer-Reported Betaine HCL Benefits

With an average customer rating of 4.5 out of 5 stars, Betaine Hydrochloride (Betaine HCL) has earned a strong reputation among users seeking relief from digestive discomfort, acid reflux, nutrient malabsorption, and low stomach acid symptoms. Many individuals who turned to this supplement did so after exhausting conventional options like proton pump inhibitors, prescription antacids, or restrictive diets, with limited or temporary results. In contrast, Betaine HCL has provided lasting digestive support for a wide range of users, from those dealing with acid reflux or bloating, to individuals navigating more complex conditions such as Hashimoto's, GERD, SIBO, or post-gallbladder removal symptoms.

The reviews reveal that users are not only finding symptom relief but also gaining a deeper understanding of how low stomach acid may have been the root cause of their discomfort. For many, this supplement became a gateway to reclaiming not just digestive comfort, but quality of life.

Use Case Patterns Observed

The most consistent use case among reviewers was digestive discomfort related to protein-rich meals or high-fat diets. People following dietary patterns like Paleo, Carnivore, or Keto frequently reported heaviness, bloating, or indigestion after eating, which significantly improved once Betaine HCL was introduced.

A large number of users came to the supplement after struggling with acid reflux, often for years. Many had been prescribed antacids or proton pump inhibitors and later realized their symptoms might stem from low stomach acid rather than excess. For these individuals, Betaine HCL often led to a reduction in heartburn, throat irritation, post-meal bloating, and the need for acid-suppressing medication.

Several users with autoimmune or digestive conditions, such as Hashimoto's thyroiditis, IBS, or chronic gastritis, shared that Betaine HCL became part of a broader healing approach. In these cases, it was commonly used alongside digestive enzymes, probiotics, aloe vera, or L-glutamine to create a supportive internal environment.

Some reviewers reported significant emotional and functional changes in daily life, such as regaining the ability to attend social events, eat at restaurants, or travel without fear of digestive episodes. In more complex cases, users found that it took some time to determine the optimal timing and dosage for their needs, but most expressed deep gratitude once they found the right balance.

Feedback Insights

The emotional tone across reviews was striking. Users frequently described their experience with words like "miracle," "life-changing," "relief," "finally," or "I wish I had known sooner." One reviewer described it as "the best decision of my adult life," ranking it just behind marrying her spouse and moving to Hawaii. Another explained that after years of "living in horror" due to reflux and stomach pain, this supplement gave them their life back.

Many reviewers expressed frustration that the concept of low stomach acid had never been mentioned to them by any doctor, despite years of suffering. There was a sense of betrayal and amazement, frustration that no one had suggested it before, mixed with joy that they had found something that worked.

Several reviewers shared highly detailed self-experiments, outlining how they tested different dosages and timing until they found what worked best. There were mentions of needing one capsule with a snack, two or three with a meal, and adjusting based on protein content. Some noticed a difference within hours or days, while others saw gradual improvements over a few weeks.

There were also emotional breakthroughs. One person noted that they had lived for 15 years thinking they had social anxiety, only to realize that their post-meal discomfort was the real trigger. After using Betaine HCL, they attended a food festival and felt no anxiety for the first time in over a decade. Another reviewer celebrated their ability to eat foods they had avoided for years, including bread and donuts, with no discomfort, calling the supplement "a miracle."

Importantly, some users described tapering off the supplement over time, emphasizing that it was not a lifelong dependency but rather a support that helped restore the body's natural digestive function. Others were comfortable taking it long-term, confident in the benefits they experienced.

Across the board, there was a tone of empowerment: users felt more in control of their digestion, their food choices, and their daily life.

Most Reported Benefits from Review Analysis

Thousands of individuals have turned to Betaine HCL in search of relief from long-standing digestive concerns, including acid reflux, bloating, and sluggish digestion. With an average customer satisfaction rating of 4.5 out of 5 stars, Betaine HCL continues to gain recognition for its ability to restore healthy stomach acid levels, enhance nutrient absorption, and provide comfort where traditional medications may have fallen short.

Our review analysis reveals consistent patterns in what people report as their most meaningful outcomes. Whether users were dealing with acid reflux triggered by protein-heavy meals or discomfort linked to low stomach acid, many found that Betaine HCL helped them reclaim a sense of normalcy and freedom around food. For some, the change was dramatic, transforming years of fear and discomfort into confident eating and restored energy.

The data below summarizes the most frequently cited benefits among positive reviews. Each percentage represents how often a specific outcome was mentioned. While experiences vary, a higher percentage indicates that a particular benefit was especially common among those who found the supplement effective.

Below is a summary table of Betaine HCL's top benefits as reported by customers:

Benefit	**%**	**Explanation**
Acid Reflux and Heartburn Relief	30%	Reported relief from reflux symptoms, throat discomfort, and nighttime burning.
Digestion Support	23%	Many noted smoother digestion, less post-meal discomfort, and better food tolerance.
Stomach Acid Balance	22%	Helped restore proper acidity for those with suspected low stomach acid.
Bloating Reduction	9%	Users described feeling lighter, with less gas and digestive heaviness.

Benefit	%	Explanation
Gut Health Support	6%	Supported microbial balance and reduced symptoms of gut dysbiosis.

How to Use This Table

This table highlights the most commonly reported benefits among users who had positive experiences with Betaine HCL. If you are experiencing similar symptoms, these patterns may help guide your expectations. For example, if your main concern is acid reflux, the data shows that a significant portion of users with that issue found relief. However, as with any supplement, individual results can vary based on underlying health conditions, diet, and dosage. Consider this table a starting point as you explore whether Betaine HCL aligns with your needs and always speak with a qualified healthcare provider before making changes to your regimen.

Application of Betaine HCL

Adding Betaine HCL to your daily regimen is straightforward but requires thoughtful integration to ensure maximum benefit. Start with a low dose, such as 300–500 mg, taken at the beginning of your largest or most problematic meal. Gradually increase the dosage until you feel improved digestion and relief from bloating or heaviness. If a warming sensation occurs in the stomach, reduce the dose slightly. Always follow product instructions or consult a healthcare professional to avoid overuse.

Betaine HCL pairs well with enzyme-rich supplements, such as beef organ capsules, as it creates an optimal digestive environment for these enzymes to function effectively. This synergy enhances protein and nutrient absorption, supporting overall digestive health.

Precautions and Safety

While Betaine HCL is generally safe when used appropriately, individuals with a history of ulcers, gastritis, or other digestive conditions should consult a healthcare provider before use. Monitor your body's response closely. If you experience discomfort or adverse effects, adjust the dosage or discontinue use under professional guidance.

By restoring balance to stomach acidity, Betaine HCL addresses a wide range of digestive concerns, making it a powerful addition to your self-care routine. It supports nutrient absorption, protects gut health, and relieves discomfort, empowering you to enjoy meals and optimize your overall well-being.

Pancreatin

Pancreatin is a powerful digestive support compound that provides a blend of naturally occurring enzymes extracted from the pancreas of healthy animals, most commonly pigs or cows. This supplement typically contains three core digestive enzymes: protease for breaking down proteins, lipase for fats, and amylase for carbohydrates. By closely mimicking the enzymes your own pancreas would produce, pancreatin can provide direct, practical support for individuals who struggle with digestive function.

In a healthy digestive system, the pancreas secretes these enzymes in response to meals. However, many factors, such as age, chronic stress, certain medications, or health conditions, can impair the body's natural enzyme production. This can lead to incomplete digestion, nutrient malabsorption, and uncomfortable symptoms such as bloating, gas, heaviness after meals, or stool irregularities. In some cases, people may not even realize their discomfort is related to poor enzyme activity until they begin supplementing and notice a difference.

Pancreatin is often recommended for individuals with difficulty digesting fatty or protein-rich meals, or for those with signs of pancreatic insufficiency. It may be especially helpful after gallbladder removal or during periods of digestive stress when enzyme production is low. By supplying these critical enzymes in a concentrated form, pancreatin helps relieve the digestive burden and supports more complete nutrient breakdown and absorption.

Science-Informed Pancreatin Benefits

Enhances Protein Digestion

One of the primary functions of pancreatin is to assist in the breakdown of dietary protein. It contains the enzyme protease, which helps convert complex proteins into absorbable amino acids. These amino acids are essential for maintaining healthy muscle tissue, supporting immune function, and enabling cellular repair. For individuals with low pancreatic enzyme activity, protein-rich meals such as meat or eggs can be difficult to digest, often resulting in a sensation of heaviness, bloating, or incomplete digestion. Scientific studies have demonstrated that protease supplementation can enhance protein metabolism, leading to improved digestive comfort and better nutrient absorption.

Supports Fat Digestion and Absorption

Pancreatin also contains lipase, the enzyme responsible for breaking down fats into fatty acids and glycerol. This process is critical not only for energy production but also for the proper absorption of fat-soluble vitamins including vitamins A, D, E, and K. Individuals who have had their gallbladder removed, or who produce insufficient bile, may find it especially difficult to digest fatty foods. Symptoms such as greasy stools, bloating, or cramping can indicate poor fat digestion. Clinical evidence supports the use of lipase to assist in fat breakdown, showing improvements in both digestion and the body's ability to utilize essential nutrients from dietary fats.

Aids Carbohydrate Digestion

Amylase, another key component of pancreatin, facilitates the breakdown of complex carbohydrates such as starches into simpler sugars like glucose. This step is necessary for the efficient absorption of energy from food. When carbohydrate digestion is impaired, it can lead to fermentation in the intestines, resulting in gas, bloating, and discomfort. Research supports that amylase supplementation can improve carbohydrate digestion and reduce the gastrointestinal symptoms often associated with undigested starches, especially in individuals with pancreatic insufficiency or sluggish enzyme activity.

Reduces Post-Meal Digestive Discomfort

Many people experience feelings of fullness, bloating, or indigestion after meals, particularly when consuming large quantities of protein or fat. Pancreatin supplementation has been clinically studied for its ability to ease these symptoms by supporting the body's natural digestive processes. In individuals with compromised enzyme production, studies have shown that taking pancreatin with meals can significantly reduce post-meal discomfort and enhance the overall digestive experience. By improving the breakdown of macronutrients, pancreatin may help meals feel lighter and easier to process.

Supports Individuals with Pancreatic and Gallbladder Challenges

People managing pancreatic conditions, such as enzyme insufficiency or chronic inflammation, often face significant barriers to proper digestion and nutrient absorption. Similarly, those who have undergone gallbladder removal may struggle to digest fats efficiently due to altered bile flow. In such cases, pancreatin can serve as an effective aid to support the digestive process. Evidence from clinical use and observational studies suggests that pancreatin supplementation may help alleviate digestive symptoms, reduce the frequency of loose stools, and improve the body's ability to extract nutrients from food. While not a cure, it offers a practical solution to help restore more comfortable and efficient digestion in these circumstances.

Customer-Reported Pancreatin Benefits

Pancreatin has received widespread praise from individuals facing a range of digestive challenges, particularly those related to enzyme insufficiency, pancreatitis, gallbladder removal, and undiagnosed post-meal discomfort. With an overall rating of 4.5 out of 5 from thousands of verified customers, it is often described as life-changing by those who struggled for years without answers. While it is not positioned as a cure or treatment for medical conditions, many users credit Pancreatin with helping them feel like themselves again, often after years of pain, bloating, or digestive disruption that had not responded to other interventions. These enzymes appear to make a noticeable difference in daily quality of life, allowing users to enjoy meals again without fear or discomfort.

Use Case Patterns Observed

A majority of users turned to Pancreatin after facing unresolved digestive issues, especially following pancreatitis, gallbladder removal, or long-term bloating and irregular stools. Many had been prescribed expensive enzyme medications, such as Creon, or experimented with a variety of other remedies without lasting results. Some had formal diagnoses of Exocrine Pancreatic Insufficiency (EPI), while others self-identified their condition after years of symptoms like undigested food, steatorrhea, or painful gas. A large number of users shared that they had been living with bloating, rapid digestion, floating or pale stools, or post-meal discomfort for months or years, often with no clear cause found by their doctors. Others, including those managing diabetes or post-surgical recovery, discovered that

Pancreatin supported more complete digestion and better energy levels throughout the day. Notably, the supplement was also widely used for dogs with pancreatic insufficiency, with owners reporting improvements in weight gain, stool quality, and vitality.

Feedback Insights

The emotional tone across user feedback is one of deep relief, often mixed with frustration that they did not discover Pancreatin sooner. Many describe it as a "quality of life saver," expressing amazement at how quickly symptoms like bloating, stomach pain, or urgency after meals improved, sometimes within just a day or two. Several users shared stories of years spent chasing a diagnosis, trying prescriptions that failed, or being dismissed by healthcare providers who did not mention enzymes as an option. They reported feeling empowered after researching their own symptoms, trying Pancreatin, and finally experiencing digestive comfort for the first time in years.

One reviewer who had suffered from chronic pancreatitis said these enzymes "changed my life" and described how their meals no longer triggered pain. Another noted the ability to enjoy normal food again without fear or urgency, saying, "It's not just a supplement, it gave me my life back." Even those without a formal diagnosis found significant benefits, with one person explaining that they "could finally eat dinner without lying awake all night with stomach pain." Others celebrated small but meaningful wins, like "not being afraid to leave the house" or "finally feeling normal after meals." For pet owners, the feedback was equally heartfelt, with comments about rescued energy, regained weight, and longer life for their beloved animals.

Overall, the reviews reflect a collective sense of hope, gratitude, and empowerment. People consistently describe Pancreatin as the missing link in their digestive routine, bringing back ease, confidence, and enjoyment to everyday life.

Most Reported Benefits from Review Analysis

Pancreatin has earned consistently high satisfaction from individuals navigating digestive discomfort, enzyme insufficiency, or post-meal challenges. With a customer rating of 4.5 out of 5, many users describe noticeable improvements in digestion, reduced bloating and gas, and an overall sense of digestive ease, especially when consuming meals that are high in protein or fat. While results may vary, these insights reflect real-world experiences shared by people seeking a solution that helps them feel more comfortable after eating.

To better understand which benefits stood out most to users, we analyzed thousands of positive reviews and tracked how often certain themes were mentioned. The percentages below represent the frequency with which a benefit was reported among those who had a positive outcome. A higher percentage suggests that if you have a similar concern, you may be more likely to experience that benefit as well.

For example, if 64 percent of reviewers noted better digestion, it means many individuals found that Pancreatin helped them break down meals more easily and reduced the discomfort they previously experienced after eating.

Below is a summary of Pancreatin's top benefits as reported by customers:

Benefit	%	Explanation
Digestion support	64%	Most users reported improved digestion, greater comfort after eating, and easier breakdown of fats, proteins, and carbs.

Benefit	%	Explanation
Gas reduction	19%	Many experienced less gas and digestive pressure, particularly after high-protein or rich meals.
Bloating relief	8%	Users noted a reduction in bloating and post-meal heaviness, allowing for greater comfort and confidence.
Energy boost	6%	Some reported increased daily energy, which may be related to more efficient nutrient use from better digestion.
Nutrient absorption	3%	A few users observed improvements in how their body responded to food, suggesting better nutrient uptake.

How to Use This Table

This table is designed to help you recognize which benefits other users most commonly noticed while using Pancreatin. If your primary concern is difficulty digesting meals or discomfort after eating, you'll see that many users experienced relief in these areas. However, as with any supplement, results can vary from person to person. Some found that benefits appeared within a few days, while others reported more gradual improvement over time.

Pancreatin works best when paired with mindful eating habits, appropriate dosing, and an awareness of how different meals may impact your digestive response. While it is not a substitute for medical care, it can be a helpful addition to your digestive support routine, especially if you've been managing enzyme insufficiency or recovering from pancreatic or gallbladder challenges

Plant-based Digestive Enzymes

Plant-based digestive enzymes offer a natural and gentle way to support the body's ability to break down food and absorb nutrients. Derived from fruits and plant sources like pineapple, papaya, and fermented fungi, these enzymes are commonly used by individuals seeking to ease digestive discomfort, particularly after heavy meals or when eating foods that are difficult to digest.

Unlike pancreatic enzymes that are animal-derived, plant-based enzymes are often favored by those following vegetarian or vegan lifestyles and by those with sensitivities to animal-based products. They function across a broader pH range in the digestive tract, which means they can begin acting as soon as food enters the stomach and continue to support digestion throughout the small intestine.

People turn to plant-based enzymes for many reasons: occasional bloating, gas, or heaviness after meals; support for breaking down proteins, fats, and carbohydrates; or general digestive wellness. Many also find these enzymes helpful during periods of stress or travel, when digestion can be less efficient. For those seeking a plant-derived solution to everyday digestive support, these enzymes offer a convenient, widely available option that can fit seamlessly into a whole-food, health-conscious lifestyle.

Science-Informed Plant-based Digestive Enzymes Benefits

Enhances protein digestion

Plant-based digestive enzyme blends commonly include fungal-derived protease, bromelain extracted from pineapple, and papain from papaya. These enzymes assist in breaking down dietary proteins into amino acids, which are essential for building and repairing tissues. This enzymatic support can be especially beneficial for individuals on high-protein or plant-based diets who may experience occasional bloating or digestive sluggishness when consuming large or complex protein-rich meals.

Supports fat digestion and absorption

Fungal-sourced lipase plays a critical role in breaking down dietary fats into fatty acids and glycerol, both of which are essential for energy production and the absorption of fat-soluble vitamins such as A, D, E, and K. Research indicates that lipase supplementation can improve fat digestion in individuals with gallbladder challenges or those consuming high-fat meals, enhancing nutrient availability and post-meal comfort.

Aids carbohydrate and fiber digestion

Many plant-based enzyme formulations include fungal-derived amylase, which helps convert complex carbohydrates into absorbable simple sugars. These blends often contain cellulase as well, an enzyme that helps break down plant fibers that are otherwise difficult for the human digestive system to process on its own. This combination may be particularly helpful for individuals following plant-heavy or high-fiber diets, who often report gas or bloating from undigested carbohydrates or fiber.

Reduces post-meal bloating and indigestion

Plant-based digestive enzyme supplements have been associated with reduced bloating, gas, and general digestive discomfort after meals. These benefits are believed to result from improved food breakdown and decreased fermentation in the gut. Studies suggest that fungal-based enzymes help support smoother digestion, especially when meals include a mix of proteins, fats, carbohydrates, and fiber-rich ingredients.

Helps individuals with food sensitivities

Many plant-based enzyme formulas include lactase, which aids in breaking down lactose, the sugar found in dairy products. This may provide support for individuals with occasional lactose sensitivity. Some blends also contain glucoamylase, an enzyme that helps break down starches and certain complex sugars that may contribute to digestive discomfort in sensitive individuals. While these enzymes do not replace medical treatment for food allergies or serious intolerances, they may support those with mild sensitivities in improving post-meal tolerance.

Customer-Reported Benefits of Plant-based Digestive Enzymes

Digestive discomfort can take many forms, bloating, gas, heaviness, or trouble with specific foods, and for many people, plant-based digestive enzymes have made a noticeable difference. With an average satisfaction rating of 4.5 out of 5, users consistently describe improvements in how they feel after meals, particularly when eating fiber-rich, high-protein, or carbohydrate-heavy foods. These enzyme supplements are especially appreciated for being gentle, effective, and versatile, often delivering relief when other options fall short. For many users, they have become a daily wellness essential.

Use Case Patterns Observed

The majority of users turned to plant-based digestive enzymes in response to persistent digestive issues, especially bloating, poor digestion of certain foods, and post-meal heaviness. Many were dealing with food sensitivities, high-fiber or plant-based diets, or conditions like IBS, GERD, or enzyme insufficiency. A significant number reported gallbladder removal, pancreatic challenges, or low enzyme production as their motivating factor. For some, these enzymes offered a more natural alternative to prescription medications or provided added support when traditional options failed to bring relief.

In particular, individuals who struggled to digest raw vegetables, gluten, dairy, or legumes found these supplements helped reduce discomfort and made meals more enjoyable. Many users on vegetarian or vegan diets reported these enzymes helped balance the effects of high plant fiber, while others appreciated the added support when consuming cooked or processed meals. A smaller group mentioned they used these enzymes as part of broader healing protocols for more complex gastrointestinal conditions.

Feedback Insights

The tone of user feedback is overwhelmingly positive, with many describing these enzymes as a “game changer,” “life saver,” or “one of the best supplements I’ve ever tried.” Users often expressed a sense of relief after trying many other options without success. Several reviewers noted that they had “tried everything” and were surprised by how quickly and consistently these enzymes improved their symptoms. A common theme is the return to normal, feeling more comfortable, less bloated, and able to enjoy foods that used to trigger discomfort.

Users with chronic bloating frequently mentioned how their midsection felt less swollen or "deflated," and many celebrated the disappearance of gas, heaviness, or unpredictable bathroom issues. Some reviewers described noticeable improvements in energy and appetite, which they attributed to better nutrient absorption and reduced digestive strain. Others shared emotional stories about regaining control over their diet or being able to enjoy meals with family again without fear or discomfort. Across the board, users appreciated the affordability, ease of use, and versatility of these supplements.

Most Reported Benefits from Review Analysis

Plant-based digestive enzyme supplements have earned consistent praise for their ability to improve digestive ease, reduce discomfort, and support everyday gut health. With an average customer satisfaction rating of 4.5 out of 5, many users share that these enzymes have helped them enjoy meals more fully and recover from food-related discomfort more quickly. For those dealing with bloating, sluggish digestion, or difficulty breaking down complex meals, these enzymes are often described as a reliable and gentle solution.

Our analysis of thousands of verified customer reviews identified the most commonly reported benefits. The percentages reflect how often each benefit was mentioned among users who shared a positive experience. A higher percentage suggests that if you have similar concerns, you may be more likely to experience that benefit as well.

For example, if 50 percent of users mentioned improved digestion, it means that half of all satisfied users noticed easier food breakdown, reduced digestive strain, and greater comfort after meals when using plant-based digestive enzymes.

Below is a summary of Plant-based Digestive Enzymes' top benefits as reported by customers:

Benefit	%	Explanation
Digestion support	50%	Many users report noticeably easier digestion, less meal-related heaviness, and better nutrient breakdown.
Gas reduction	26%	Helps reduce uncomfortable gas, particularly after meals high in fiber, legumes, or raw vegetables.
Bloating relief	19%	Users frequently describe a visible and physical reduction in bloating and fullness.
Energy boost	3%	A small but meaningful group of users noted improved energy, likely due to better nutrient absorption.
Stomach discomfort relief	3%	Some users experience less irritation, sensitivity, or post-meal unease with regular use.

How to Use This Table

This summary offers a helpful snapshot of how real users benefit from plant-based digestive enzymes. While not every benefit applies to every person, these trends reflect common experiences among those who reported positive outcomes. If you are struggling with bloating, gas, or post-meal heaviness, especially after high-fiber or plant-heavy meals, this table can help you decide whether plant-based enzymes are a good match for your needs. Individual responses can vary, so it may take some experimentation with timing or dosage to find what works best for your body.

Pancreatin vs Plant-based Enzymes

Key Differences of Pancreatin vs Plant-based Digestive Enzymes in Customer-Reported Benefits

Feature	Pancreatin	Plant-based Enzymes
Main Benefit Focus	Digestion of high-fat and high-protein meals	General gut health, bloating, and fiber digestion
Top Issues Addressed	Gas, bloating, and digestion issues related to fat and protein intake	Bloating, gas, fiber digestion, and lactose intolerance
Most Likely Users	People with pancreatic insufficiency, gallbladder issues, or high-fat diets	People with plant-heavy diets, dairy sensitivities, or general digestion issues
Energy & Nutrient Absorption Mentions	Reported, but secondary	Less frequently mentioned

The best enzyme supplement depends on individual digestive needs and dietary habits. Pancreatin is best for high-protein, high-fat diets and pancreatic/gallbladder support. Plant-based enzymes are ideal for general digestion support, plant-heavy diets, or dairy intolerance.

By incorporating the right digestive enzyme supplement, you can improve nutrient absorption, reduce digestive discomfort, and optimize gut health.

Vitamin D

Multivitamins and Whole-Food Nutrition

Multivitamins are often seen as a convenient way to fill nutritional gaps, but convenience does not always equal effectiveness. The *Medicine-Free, Illness-Free Series* and the HOPED Protocol emphasize a different approach, one rooted in nature, not factories. Rather than relying on synthetic blends of isolated nutrients, this philosophy encourages obtaining nourishment from whole-food-based sources that the body recognizes and utilizes more efficiently.

Many commercial multivitamins are produced using synthetic or fractionated nutrients. These lack the natural co-factors, enzymes, and biological synergy found in real food. Without these elements, the body may struggle to absorb or properly use the nutrients. In some cases, excessive intake of certain isolated vitamins from multivitamins can even lead to imbalances or unwanted effects.

By contrast, whole-food-based options such as herbal remedies, functional mushrooms, animal organ supplements, and nutrient-dense meals offer vitamins and minerals in forms the body has evolved to process. These sources deliver nutrients in balance with their natural co-factors, supporting more effective absorption and function.

Herbs offer a wide spectrum of naturally occurring vitamins, minerals, and antioxidants that help maintain vitality and support the body's internal systems.

Medicinal mushrooms like Reishi, Turkey Tail, and Lion's Mane contribute valuable compounds including B vitamins, beta-glucans, and other nutrients that support resilience.

Animal organ supplements, particularly from grass-fed beef liver, provide concentrated, highly bioavailable sources of vitamin A, iron, B-complex vitamins, and trace minerals.

These natural, food-derived options are discussed in depth throughout the other books in this series. In this chapter, however, we turn our attention to one specific nutrient that often requires direct supplementation—Vitamin D.

Vitamin D: The Essential Vitamin You Can't Ignore

Vitamin D holds a unique place among nutrients because it is not primarily obtained through food. Instead, our bodies are designed to produce it when skin is exposed to sunlight. Despite this built-in system, Vitamin D deficiency has become widespread, affecting people across different regions, lifestyles, and age groups.

What makes Vitamin D essential is not just its widespread deficiency, but its powerful influence on energy levels, immune health, bone strength, mental clarity, and cardiovascular support. Within the HOPED Protocol, it plays a foundational role in restoring balance where modern life often creates gaps.

If natural production through sun exposure is inconsistent or unavailable, targeted supplementation becomes not only helpful but often necessary. The following sections will explain why deficiency is so prevalent and what you can do to naturally and effectively support your Vitamin D levels year-round.

Why Is Vitamin D Deficiency So Common?

Although the body is equipped to produce Vitamin D from sunlight, modern lifestyles have made this natural process increasingly unreliable. People spend more time indoors than ever, working, commuting, and relaxing, which limits the skin's exposure to the ultraviolet B (UVB) rays required for Vitamin D synthesis. Even those who venture outside often use sunscreen, which is essential for skin protection but also blocks the UVB rays that trigger Vitamin D production.

Geography is another major factor. Individuals living in northern regions, where daylight hours are shorter and sun angles are lower during winter, may be unable to produce enough Vitamin D for several months each year.

Skin pigmentation plays a role as well. People with darker skin have more melanin, which naturally filters UVB rays and reduces Vitamin D production. This means that individuals with deeper skin tones may need more sun exposure to maintain adequate levels.

As we age, our skin becomes less efficient at synthesizing Vitamin D, and older adults often spend even less time outdoors. On top of that, very few foods naturally provide meaningful amounts of Vitamin D. While fatty fish, liver, and egg yolks are notable sources, they are not commonly consumed in sufficient quantity to close the gap.

With so many overlapping factors at play, it's clear why supplementation has become a practical and often necessary solution for maintaining healthy Vitamin D status, particularly during the winter months or in cases of limited sun exposure.

Sunlight: Your Most Natural Source of Vitamin D

The most efficient and natural way for the body to produce Vitamin D is through exposure to sunlight. When UVB rays strike the skin, they convert a form of cholesterol into Vitamin D3, which is then activated by the liver and kidneys to support vital processes throughout the body.

To support healthy levels, short periods of sun exposure, generally about 10 to 30 minutes on areas like the arms, legs, and face, can be effective a few times per week. The amount needed varies depending on factors such as time of day, season, geographic location, and individual skin tone. People with darker skin or those living in northern regions may require longer exposure to generate similar benefits.

For safety, it's best to seek sun exposure during non-peak hours and limit duration to avoid skin damage. Some experts recommend allowing brief exposure before applying sunscreen, especially when aiming to support Vitamin D production, as sunscreen blocks UVB rays. However, caution should always be exercised, and sunburn must be avoided.

If regular sun exposure is not practical due to climate, season, or personal risk factors, high-quality Vitamin D supplementation can help bridge the gap, ensuring your body receives the support it needs without relying solely on sunshine.

Science-Informed Vitamin D Benefits

Vitamin D is a fat-soluble nutrient with far-reaching influence across multiple body systems. Though traditionally known for its role in bone health, modern research has revealed its importance in supporting immune balance, mental clarity, cardiovascular function, and metabolic processes. The body produces Vitamin D through sunlight exposure, but supplementation is often necessary due to lifestyle and environmental factors that limit sun access. Below are the key science-informed benefits of Vitamin D.

Supports Bone Strength and Calcium Utilization

Vitamin D plays a central role in calcium and phosphorus balance, helping the body absorb and retain these minerals to support bone density and skeletal integrity. It promotes the activity of osteoblasts, the cells responsible for building bone tissue, and helps maintain bone mineralization over time. Without adequate Vitamin D, calcium absorption declines, increasing the risk of weakened bones. Research supports its role in promoting bone health across all ages and maintaining structural strength in older adults.

Promotes a Balanced Immune Response

Immune cells such as macrophages and T cells contain Vitamin D receptors, allowing this nutrient to influence immune activity. Studies show that Vitamin D plays a role in modulating both the innate and adaptive branches of the immune system, helping the body respond appropriately to pathogens while minimizing overactive inflammatory responses. Adequate levels of Vitamin D are associated with better outcomes during respiratory illnesses and may contribute to a more balanced immune defense throughout the year.

Contributes to Mood Stability and Cognitive Function

Vitamin D is involved in neurological health through its impact on neurotransmitter activity, including the synthesis of serotonin, a key regulator of mood and emotional resilience. Low levels of Vitamin D have been observed in individuals experiencing low mood, cognitive decline, or seasonal affective changes. Some studies suggest a link between healthy Vitamin D status and improved mental clarity, memory retention, and emotional balance.

Supports Cardiovascular Function

Vitamin D contributes to heart health by influencing vascular tone, supporting endothelial cell function, and helping regulate blood pressure. It also plays a role in calcium metabolism, which can impact arterial health and reduce calcification risk. While ongoing research is examining the full scope of its cardiovascular benefits, maintaining adequate Vitamin D levels is considered an important factor for overall vascular health and systemic inflammation balance.

Assists in Blood Sugar Regulation

Emerging evidence suggests that Vitamin D may support insulin sensitivity and glucose metabolism. It appears to play a role in how the body processes carbohydrates, helping maintain stable blood sugar levels. Some studies associate lower Vitamin D levels with an increased risk of metabolic imbalance, including challenges related to weight regulation and energy utilization.

Supports Skin Wellness and Cellular Repair

Vitamin D contributes to skin renewal by influencing the function and differentiation of keratinocytes, the primary cells found in the outer layer of the skin. It also plays a role in managing localized inflammation and supporting the skin's natural barrier function. Research suggests it may be helpful for maintaining healthy skin tone and integrity, particularly in individuals with dry, sensitive, or reactive skin.

Customer-Reported Vitamin D Benefits

Vitamin D is one of the most widely used supplements in the world, and for good reason. Thousands of users turn to Vitamin D3 to help restore their energy, improve their mood, support immunity, and address symptoms that stem from low or suboptimal levels. While Vitamin D is often categorized as a nutrient, many users describe it as a life-changing daily essential that noticeably enhances how they feel, think, and function.

In analyzing a broad range of verified reviews, a few patterns become clear: people are using Vitamin D not just for long-term maintenance, but because they feel a real, tangible difference. From lifting the fog of fatigue to strengthening immune resilience, the feedback reflects how this single nutrient has become a foundational part of health routines for millions, especially those who don't get enough sun exposure or have absorption challenges. What follows is a closer look at how and why people are using Vitamin D, and what kinds of results they are reporting.

Use Case Patterns Observed

Vitamin D is commonly used to address deficiency or insufficiency, often confirmed through bloodwork, or to maintain healthy levels year-round. Individuals most likely to use this supplement include those with darker skin tones, limited sun exposure, autoimmune conditions, or digestive issues that impact nutrient absorption. Others use it preventively to support immune function, enhance bone strength, regulate mood, or improve energy.

Reviewers frequently note that their doctor recommended Vitamin D supplementation, especially when symptoms like fatigue, low mood, frequent illness, or muscle aches were present. Some users take Vitamin D on its own, while many combine it with magnesium, Vitamin K2, or omega-3s for enhanced synergy. Pregnant women, older adults, and those recovering from illness or surgery also report including Vitamin D as part of their targeted wellness plan.

Feedback Insights

The most consistent and emotionally resonant feedback centers around energy and mood. Many users describe starting out feeling exhausted, low on motivation, or emotionally flat, especially during colder seasons. After supplementing with Vitamin D, they report feeling "brighter," "more stable," and "mentally clearer," often within the first one to two weeks. For some, the change was so significant that they compared it to "waking up fully for the first time in months."

Mood-related feedback includes reduced anxiety, better emotional balance, and a decrease in seasonal blues. Several users who had considered prescription options found that Vitamin D gave them a surprisingly effective and gentle alternative. The sense of "emotional grounding" and "daylight in a bottle" is a recurring sentiment among those who had previously struggled with mood regulation or low-grade depression.

Energy improvements were also widely noted. Users reported feeling more productive during the day, experiencing fewer afternoon crashes, and sleeping more restfully at night. Some found relief from muscle soreness or stiffness, especially when their deficiency had previously gone undiagnosed. A number of reviews also mentioned immune-related benefits, such as getting sick less often or bouncing back more quickly from common colds.

Importantly, many reviewers described feeling a clear difference between high-quality Vitamin D brands and cheaper options. Those who experimented with different forms or dosages consistently emphasized the importance of absorption, noting that they could "feel the difference" with better formulations. Several reviewers even said that their symptoms returned when switching to lower-quality products, reinforcing the importance of choosing trusted, well-formulated supplements.

Together, these user experiences paint a compelling picture of why Vitamin D is a cornerstone in many health routines, and why so many people continue to take it year after year.

Most Reported Benefits from Review Analysis

Vitamin D continues to receive strong praise from users for its impact on daily energy, emotional resilience, immune strength, and physical well-being. Across thousands of reviews, people consistently describe a noticeable difference in how they feel once their Vitamin D levels are supported, often calling it a foundational supplement they wish they had discovered sooner. Whether taken for deficiency or general wellness, Vitamin D is widely credited with helping people regain balance, vitality, and peace of mind.

Our analysis of verified reviews highlights the most frequently reported benefits based on positive user experiences. The percentages shown below reflect how often each benefit was mentioned among those who felt the supplement made a meaningful difference. A higher percentage suggests that if you are facing similar concerns, you may be more likely to experience that benefit too.

For example, if 40 percent of reviewers reported improved immune function, this suggests a strong pattern among users who experienced fewer seasonal illnesses or stronger overall resistance after consistent use of Vitamin D.

Below is a summary of Vitamin D's top benefits as reported by customers:

Benefit	%	Explanation
Immune system support	40%	Many users reported fewer colds, faster recovery from illness, and overall improved immune resilience.
Energy boost	20%	Users noted higher daytime energy and reduced fatigue, particularly in winter or after confirmed deficiency.
Bone and joint health	20%	Reviewers highlighted better joint comfort, stronger bones, and reduced aches or stiffness.
Mood and mental clarity	13%	Many experienced improved mood, fewer depressive symptoms, and enhanced mental focus or calm.
Skin health	7%	Some users found relief from dry or irritated skin and noticed improvements in skin tone and inflammation.

How to Use This Table

This summary highlights the most common outcomes people reported after taking Vitamin D supplements. While individual responses vary, the frequency of these reported benefits can help guide your expectations. If your goals align with the experiences shown here, such as boosting immune resilience, lifting fatigue, or improving mood, you may find similar support by adding Vitamin D to your routine.

Always consult with a qualified health provider before starting any new supplement, especially if you have underlying health conditions or are taking medications. For best results, choose high-quality

Vitamin D3 products and consider pairing them with Vitamin K2 or magnesium to enhance absorption and effectiveness, as many users do.

Supporting Vitamin D Year-Round

The science and real-world experiences speak clearly: maintaining adequate Vitamin D levels can have a meaningful impact on energy, immune health, bone strength, mood, and more. But knowing its importance is only the first step. The next challenge is practical, how can you ensure your body consistently gets the Vitamin D it needs? For many people, sunlight alone is not enough, and dietary sources are limited. That's where thoughtful supplementation comes in. Whole-food-based and high-quality supplemental forms of Vitamin D can help bridge the gap. Here are some well-regarded sources:

Fish Egg Supplements

Fish eggs are a rich, natural source of Vitamin D, Omega-3 fatty acids, and other essential nutrients. Available in capsule form, fish egg supplements offer a concentrated, whole-food-based option for those seeking to support brain function, skin health, and overall vitality without relying on more expensive foods like fresh caviar.

Cod Liver Oil

A traditional and trusted source of Vitamin D, cod liver oil also contains Omega-3 fatty acids and naturally occurring Vitamin A. Just one or two teaspoons a day of high-quality cod liver oil can provide meaningful levels of these fat-soluble nutrients. When selecting a product, it is important to ensure it has been properly purified to remove environmental contaminants.

Algal Oil

Ideal for those who follow vegetarian or vegan lifestyles, algal oil offers a plant-based form of Vitamin D3. Derived from marine algae, it also contains Omega-3s and is available in easy-to-use capsule form. Algal oil is a sustainable and effective way to supplement Vitamin D for those avoiding animal-based products.

High-Quality Vitamin D3 Supplements from Animal Sources

Vitamin D3 (cholecalciferol) is the preferred form for maintaining healthy levels in the body. Supplements made from animal-derived lanolin (from sheep's wool) are among the most commonly used. Most high-quality Vitamin D3 supplements offer dosages ranging from 1,000 IU to 4,000 IU per day. For many individuals, 2,000 IU is a typical daily amount, although needs may vary. It is always wise to follow the label or consult a healthcare professional to determine what dosage is right for you.

HOPED for Everyday Health Goals

Earlier chapters introduced each supplement within the HOPED Protocol individually, exploring their science-informed benefits and customer-reported results. This chapter takes a more practical approach: it organizes those insights by everyday health goals, making it easier for you to look up which supplements are most commonly used to support specific areas such as energy, immunity, digestion, focus, sleep, or stress resilience.

The percentages listed next to each solution come from our *Most Reported Benefits from Review Analysis*, which examines real-world customer feedback to identify the most frequently mentioned effects for each supplement. These figures offer a snapshot of how people are using these products in practice, and which benefits tend to stand out most often in their experiences.

This chapter is not a replacement for the in-depth profiles provided earlier. Instead, it serves as a quick-reference guide, designed for those who want to connect specific wellness needs with the supplements most often chosen to support them. It brings together both scientific rationale and user insight in a format that is clear, actionable, and easy to revisit.

As always, this content is intended for educational purposes only. It is not meant to diagnose, treat, cure, or prevent any disease. While many users report positive outcomes, individual results may vary depending on your overall health, lifestyle, supplement quality, and consistency of use.

This summary chapter is here to support your ongoing wellness journey, helping you make informed, thoughtful decisions, ideally in partnership with your qualified healthcare provider.

Bone Health

Vitamin D (20%) – Frequently praised for supporting bone strength, flexibility, and overall skeletal comfort.

Scientific perspective: Vitamin D plays a central role in calcium absorption and supports proper bone mineralization, contributing to long-term skeletal maintenance.

Cardiovascular Support

CoQ10 (49%) – Widely used to support cardiovascular vitality and daily stamina.

Scientific perspective: CoQ10 is essential for ATP production, particularly in heart tissue, and may help maintain normal cardiovascular energy levels.

Resveratrol (28%) – Supports circulation and overall heart wellness.

Scientific perspective: This polyphenol has antioxidant properties and may help maintain endothelial health and vascular flexibility.

Fish Oil (16%) – Commonly taken to support heart function and lipid balance.

Scientific perspective: EPA and DHA are omega-3 fatty acids shown to influence cardiovascular biomarkers and help maintain a healthy inflammatory response.

Fish Eggs (10%) – Used to support circulation and heart performance.

Scientific perspective: A concentrated source of EPA, DHA, and phospholipids, fish eggs may help maintain cardiovascular resilience and vascular health.

Cognitive Health

Fish Eggs (22%) – Users frequently report sharper thinking and improved memory recall.

Scientific perspective: Rich in omega-3s and phospholipids, fish eggs help support healthy neuronal structure and brain cell signaling.

Fish Oil (13%) – Chosen to support cognitive sharpness and mental focus.

Scientific perspective: DHA, a key component of fish oil, is vital for brain cell membrane integrity and is linked to healthy cognitive performance.

Resveratrol (10%) – Supports mental clarity and concentration.

Scientific perspective: Known for its antioxidant activity, resveratrol may help maintain cerebral blood flow and protect brain cells from oxidative stress.

Vitamin D (13%) – Used to support mood balance and mental clarity.

Scientific perspective: Vitamin D receptors in the brain may influence neurotransmitter activity and emotional well-being.

Shilajit (8%) – Reported to enhance overall clarity and productivity.

Scientific perspective: Shilajit contains fulvic acid and trace minerals that may support mitochondrial function and cellular energy in brain tissue.

Digestive Health

Psyllium Husk (80%) – Commonly used to support bowel regularity and ease constipation, contributing to overall digestive comfort.

Scientific perspective: As a rich source of soluble fiber, psyllium absorbs water to form bulk in the intestines, supporting smoother bowel movements and promoting the growth of beneficial gut bacteria.

Pancreatin (91%) – Frequently praised for easing post-meal heaviness, discomfort, and supporting efficient digestion.

Scientific perspective: Pancreatin contains a blend of key digestive enzymes including amylase, protease, and lipase, which aid in the breakdown of carbohydrates, proteins, and fats.

Plant-Based Digestive Enzymes (69%) – Often selected to improve food breakdown and reduce bloating and gas.

Scientific perspective: These enzymes help digest a range of macronutrients and may support digestive comfort, particularly in those with plant-heavy or high-fiber diets.

Gut Probiotics (58%) – Trusted for promoting healthy digestion and supporting regularity.

Scientific perspective: A diverse and balanced gut microbiome is essential for nutrient absorption, immune defense, and optimal gastrointestinal function.

Betaine HCL (45%) – Chosen to support stomach acid levels and enhance protein digestion.

Scientific perspective: Adequate hydrochloric acid is critical for the initial stages of digestion and for creating an environment that supports nutrient absorption and microbial balance.

Betaine HCL (30%) – Used to relieve occasional acid reflux and heartburn.

Scientific perspective: Restoring stomach acidity can support digestive function and help prevent the backflow of stomach contents that contribute to discomfort.

Oral Health

Oral Probiotics (33%) – Frequently reported to promote overall oral wellness, including fresher breath and cleaner-feeling teeth.

Scientific perspective: Certain probiotic strains support microbial balance in the mouth, helping to maintain oral hygiene and limit the growth of harmful bacteria.

Oral Probiotics (27%) – Often used to address unpleasant breath.

Scientific perspective: By reducing odor-producing bacteria, probiotics can help support fresher breath through natural microbial balancing.

Oral Probiotics (20%) – Chosen to support healthy gums and ease occasional gum discomfort.

Scientific perspective: Select probiotic strains may help reduce oral inflammation and support a balanced environment that promotes gum health.

Oral Probiotics (12%) – Used to help maintain healthy teeth and reduce the risk of plaque buildup.

Scientific perspective: Beneficial bacteria may compete with cavity-causing organisms, supporting a more protective oral environment.

Oral Probiotics (7%) – Reported to support throat and sinus comfort.

Scientific perspective: Establishing a healthy probiotic presence in the upper airway may help reduce colonization of unwanted microbes in the mouth and sinuses.

Energy and Fatigue

Shilajit (44%) – Frequently reported to improve daily energy, stamina, and overall vitality.

Scientific perspective: Shilajit contains fulvic acid and trace minerals that may support mitochondrial efficiency, contributing to more consistent energy production at the cellular level.

Fish Eggs (37%) – Chosen by many for enhanced physical resilience and steady energy.

Scientific perspective: Rich in omega-3s, phospholipids, and essential micronutrients, fish eggs help fuel mitochondrial activity and reduce systemic inflammation, both of which support sustained energy.

CoQ10 (35%) – Used to support energy levels, especially during physical or mental fatigue.

Scientific perspective: CoQ10 plays a central role in ATP generation within the electron transport chain, helping the body produce and manage energy more efficiently.

Resveratrol (30%) – Often credited for improving endurance and reducing fatigue.

Scientific perspective: Resveratrol may enhance mitochondrial function through sirtuin activation and supports antioxidant defenses, which protect energy-producing cells from oxidative stress.

Vitamin D (20%) – Chosen to support mood, motivation, and energy levels.

Scientific perspective: Adequate Vitamin D levels help regulate mitochondrial activity, hormone balance, and inflammation, all of which contribute to a person's sense of vitality.

Immune System

Vitamin D (41%) – Many users report fewer seasonal illnesses and improved resilience.

Scientific perspective: Vitamin D plays a key role in modulating the innate and adaptive immune responses and supports healthy inflammatory balance.

Gut Probiotics (11%) – Used to support immune strength and general wellness.

Scientific perspective: A healthy gut microbiome is essential for immune function, as the majority of immune cells reside in the gastrointestinal tract.

Joint Health

Fish Oil (9%) – Selected to help with joint flexibility and morning stiffness.

Scientific perspective: EPA and DHA in fish oil support a healthy inflammatory response, which may benefit joint mobility and comfort.

Reproductive Support

Shilajit (10%) – Commonly used for support in libido and reproductive vitality.

Scientific perspective: Shilajit has long been valued in traditional systems for male reproductive support, and modern research suggests it may help optimize hormone balance and energy metabolism.

Skin Health

Resveratrol (32%) – Frequently used for skin health and appearance.

Scientific perspective: Resveratrol offers antioxidant protection and supports cellular repair pathways, promoting more youthful, resilient skin.

Fish Eggs (22%) – Chosen for improved skin hydration and elasticity.

Scientific perspective: Omega-3s and phospholipids found in fish eggs support the skin's moisture barrier, improving tone and softness from the inside out.

Fish Oil (13%) – Used to ease dryness and redness and support smoother skin.

Scientific perspective: EPA and DHA help regulate inflammation and reinforce the skin's lipid layer, which is essential for hydration and comfort.

Restful Sleep

Shilajit (13%) – Often used to promote deeper, more restful sleep.

Scientific perspective: Shilajit may help support healthy cortisol rhythms and nervous system balance, both of which influence sleep quality.

Stress Management

Shilajit (25%) – Users often describe feeling more relaxed and emotionally balanced.

Scientific perspective: Fulvic acid and trace minerals in Shilajit may influence neurotransmitter activity and help modulate the body's response to stress.

A Final Word: The Journey to Vibrant Health

As we come to the end of this guide on the HOPED Protocol, take a moment to appreciate the simplicity and strength of what you've explored. The solutions presented in this book are not about doing more; they're about doing what works. Grounded in science and validated by real-world experience, the HOPED Protocol offers a clear, natural path to restoring balance and supporting your body's core systems.

Throughout these pages, you've seen how targeted supplementation, focused on fiber, omega-3s, probiotics, enzymes, and essential vitamins, can help support digestion, immunity, energy, cardiovascular resilience, and more. These are not treatments or cures, but time-tested tools that many people find useful in optimizing how they feel and function.

One of the most powerful aspects of this approach is its flexibility. You don't need to follow a strict regimen or overhaul your life to experience meaningful results. For many, adding just one or two well-chosen supplements has led to greater energy, more comfort, or a deeper sense of well-being. The HOPED Protocol was designed to fit real life, easily, sustainably, and naturally.

Healing is not about perfection. It's about consistency, curiosity, and listening to what your body needs. Every small choice you make, whether it's taking a supplement, adjusting your diet, or supporting your microbiome, moves you closer to the health you want.

This volume is just one piece of *The Medicine-Free, Illness-Free Series*, which includes additional books on Herbal Therapy, Mushroom Therapy, Animal Organ Therapy, Amino Acid Therapy, Grounding Therapy, Detoxification, and Lifestyle. Each book is designed to offer practical, science-informed options to help you build a health routine that works for you.

May this book empower you to move forward with clarity and confidence. Your path to sustainable wellness is uniquely yours, and nature has given you everything you need to walk it well.

To explore more solutions or receive personalized guidance, visit AshiHealing.com.

About the Author

Dr. Forest Yin (Jie Yin) is a licensed acupuncturist, herbalist, and Doctor of Acupuncture and Oriental Medicine (DAOM). He serves as a professor and doctoral advisor at the University of East West Medicine (UEWM) and is the founder of Ashi Healing and Acupuncture Inc. With extensive experience in Traditional Chinese Medicine (TCM) and natural health, Dr. Yin integrates a wide range of holistic therapies, forming the foundation of *The Medicine-Free, Illness-Free Series.*

Before devoting his career fully to natural healing, Dr. Yin worked in the high-tech and financial sectors with both large corporations and fast-paced startups. These experiences gave him firsthand insight into the chronic stress and burnout common in modern life. Inspired to seek sustainable strategies for long-term wellness, he turned to the wisdom of nature and the depth of Chinese medicine.

Dr. Yin's clinical experience and ongoing research have helped shape practical wellness protocols that focus on balance, energy, and lifestyle-based health support. His work emphasizes simple, science-informed approaches that align with the body's natural rhythms and support overall resilience.

Driven by a mission to empower others, he created *The Medicine-Free, Illness-Free Series* to share accessible natural strategies that fit seamlessly into busy lives. His approach blends ancient healing principles with modern insight, helping people feel more energized, focused, and in tune with their long-term health goals.

Continue Your Wellness Journey

This book is just the beginning. True wellness is a lifelong journey, and you don't have to walk it alone. The Ashi Healing ecosystem is here to support you every step of the way with personalized guidance, nature-based solutions, and a shared mission: to help more people experience the benefits of natural health.

Personalized Virtual Consultation

If you're ready for expert guidance tailored to your specific needs, you can schedule a private virtual consultation with Dr. Forest Yin at AshiHealing.com. These one-on-one sessions offer a personalized supplement and herbal plan based on your current wellness goals, lifestyle, and health history, helping you create a sustainable path forward using time-tested, natural approaches.

In-Person Consultation and Acupuncture

If you're located in the San Francisco Bay Area, Dr. Yin also provides in-person consultations and acupuncture sessions at the University of East West Medicine (UEWM) campus in Sunnyvale, California, where he also teaches in the doctoral program for Traditional Chinese Medicine. This serene, professional setting offers a welcoming space for personalized care. All visits, virtual or in-person, can be scheduled through AshiHealing.com.

Supplement Recommendation Plans

Each wellness protocol discussed in this book has a corresponding supplement plan available on Fullscript, featuring practitioner-trusted, food-based formulas. These curated plans make it easy to take action without guesswork, offering clear, guided steps for nutritional support.

You can access them directly at:

https://us.fullscript.com/welcome/ashi-healing,

or simply start from AshiHealing.com.

Explore the Complete Book Series

This book is part of *The Medicine-Free, Illness-Free Series*, a 10-book collection designed to help you support your long-term health and vitality through natural methods. Each volume introduces a unique modality—from herbs and mushrooms to detoxification, grounding, amino acids, and more—so you can build your wellness path one step at a time.

Refer to the Series Overview chapter or visit AshiHealing.com to explore the full collection.

Support the Natural Health Movement

If this book has inspired you, and you believe more people should have access to clear, trustworthy information about natural health, consider supporting our mission.

The Ashi Healing Foundation *(AshiHealing.org)* is a nonprofit organization dedicated to public education, natural health awareness, and holistic wellness outreach. Your tax-deductible donation helps expand access to these tools and empowers more individuals to explore safe, evidence-informed approaches to well-being.

To contribute, visit AshiHealing.org and join the movement for a healthier, freer world.

Connect and Stay Inspired

Your healing journey doesn't end here.

Follow **Dr. Forest Yin** for more healing stories, tips, and inspiration:

Instagram, TikTok, YouTube, and X: @DrForestYin

Facebook: @DrForestYin1

LinkedIn: linkedin.com/in/forest-yin

Ready to Take the Next Step?

Scan the QR code below to visit AshiHealing.com, your starting point for virtual consultations, supplement plans, and more resources.

Your journey toward sustainable, natural wellness begins now.

Made in the USA
Monee, IL
08 November 2026

68007856R00114